innocent

smoothie recipe book

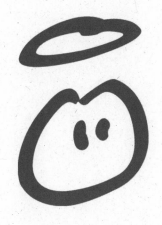

also by innocent:

little book of drinks
stay healthy, be lazy

innocent

smoothie recipe book

57½ recipes
from our kitchen to yours

FOURTH ESTATE · London

First published in Great Britain in 2006 by
Fourth Estate
An imprint of HarperCollins*Publishers*
77–85 Fulham Palace Road
London W6 8JB
www.4thestate.co.uk

5 7 9 8 6 4

The innocent wee-ometer first appeared in *Stay Healthy, Be Lazy*,
a book we wrote a couple of years ago.

Jamie Oliver's mango and ginger smoothie © Jamie Oliver 2006

A catalogue record for this book is
available from the British Library

ISBN-13 978-0-00-721376-4
ISBN-10 0-00-721376-X

Printed in Italy by Lego Spa on recycled paper

Read in your kitchen by you

thanks mum

Credits

These people made this book:

Recipes
Lucy Ede
Lucy Thomas
Nikki Elphick
Amy Hasloch
Eleanor Freeman
Sarah Oliver

Text
Dan Germain

Design
Joby Barnard
Rachel Smyth
Ed Grace
Kat Linger
Julian Humphries

Photography
Clare Shilland

Watchful eye
Dan Shrimpton
Richard Reed

Editor
Louise Haines

Assistant editor
Silvia Crompton

Home economist
Karen Taylor

Contents

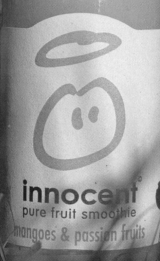

hello

We're innocent and we make smoothies. We started making smoothies in 1999, after we realised that we were eating a few too many doughnuts. So we decided to start doing something a bit healthier, and making smoothies seemed like a good idea. Seven years later and we're still doing the same thing – getting hold of the best fruit in the world, inventing new recipes and trying to avoid the doughnuts.

But a little while ago we had a thought. Perhaps it's time to write a recipe book. We did one about four years ago, when we were young and foolish, but time marches on. Since then, we've spent hundreds and maybe even thousands of hours in the kitchen inventing new drinks. We've had loads of new ideas. We've had babies and grown beards.

So now it's time to share all of the new stuff (the recipes, not the beards). On the following pages you'll find our all-time classics and our latest ideas. You'll find recipes that innocent drinkers have sent us and recipes from professional foodies, like that nice Jamie Oliver. You'll also find some other stuff that we've been thinking about that doesn't necessarily have to do with making drinks.

Anyway, we hope you enjoy making and drinking these recipes. If you've got any thoughts at all on this book or what we're doing, or you're just a bit bored and fancy a chat, we're always here. Email hello@innocentdrinks.co.uk or if you're in the neighbourhood, pop in for a smoothie.

where the money's going

It's all a bit Miss World, but we genuinely want to leave things a tiny bit better than the way we found them. First and foremost, this means that we'll always make 100% natural, healthy drinks in a responsible, sustainable manner. But it also means giving 10% of the profits from this book straight to the innocent foundation, like we do with all of our drinks.

Find out more on page 88 or check out www.innocentfoundation.org

why drinking smoothies and juices is the most important thing in the world*

Well, there's a long answer and there's a short answer.

Short answer first. Juices and smoothies are very good for you. When made properly, they're thoroughly natural, full of all of the benefits of fruit and veg. They don't contain weird additives or concentrates or chemicals, and they taste amazing.

The long answer is a bit more of a meander, and merely expands upon the short answer. You see, without wanting to sound too hippyish, the stuff that we eat and drink turns into us. Every fibre, every protein and every vitamin that we get from food and drink is used by our bodies in some way to build a bit more of us, or to repair something, or to fight a disease. If you put good stuff in, the chances of you living a longer and happier life are greater.

When it comes down to it, this is the guiding thought behind everything we do — we know that good food is lifesaving stuff, so we'll only ever make something that's good for you. But the problem with a lot of healthy stuff is that it tastes rubbish. Man cannot live on mung beans alone.

So that's why we love smoothies and juices — because they tick the healthy box and manage to taste special at the same time. They make the art of staying healthy really simple — you drink something that tastes phenomenal and find that it's actually doing you a great deal of good too.

You could look at it like this — when we're old and grey we want to look back and say that we made something that was good for people, something that helped them get to the old and grey place without too much trouble. Life's too short to waste on crisps and mechanically recovered chicken 'pieces'.

We'll drink to that.

*after remembering your nan's birthday

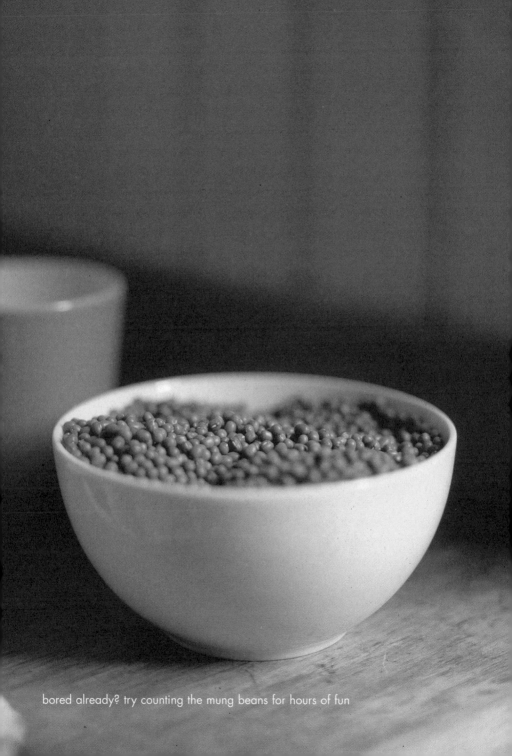

bored already? try counting the mung beans for hours of fun

do I need to buy a juicer?

This is a question we get asked a lot. There are three main bits of kit you'll need when making smoothies, and each one is used on a different type of fruit/veg:

Hard stuff (like apples and carrots) should be juiced with a juicer

Soft stuff (like berries and mangoes) should be blended in a blender

Citrus stuff (like oranges and lemons) should be squeezed with a citrus squeezer

See? That's not too tough to follow. So if you want to make everything in this book, you'll need all three bits of kit at some point – a juicer, a blender and a squeezer. However, some recipes might only require one or two of them. More about the specific kits overleaf.

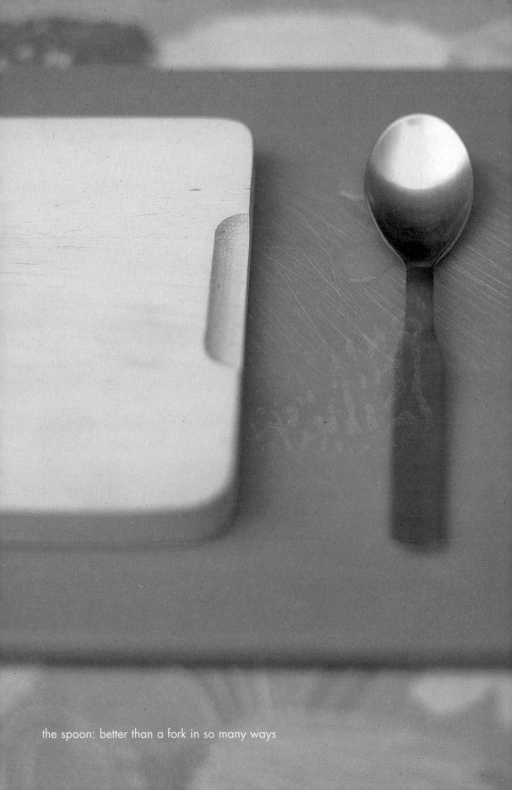

the spoon: better than a fork in so many ways

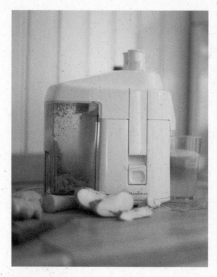
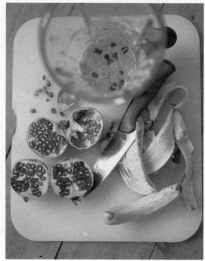

the kit

our juicer

As you can imagine, we've worked with quite a few juicers. The one we use for day-to-day juicing is the Moulinex 753. It serves us well and gets all of the juice out of apples and pears and parsnips and all of the other hard stuff. And it only cost us about £30.

Of course, you could spend a lot more on a juicer. Ours is a simple centrifugal juicer, but you can spend hundreds of pounds on masticating or hydraulic machines.

Our advice is to start off simple. Spend your money on great ingredients rather than a bit of kit you use once a month. And get a juicer that's dishwasher-friendly.

our blender

This is the rock upon which our kitchen is built. Without it, our empire would crumble. And it would be quite difficult to make drinks too. We currently use a Kenwood BL900 and we love it because...

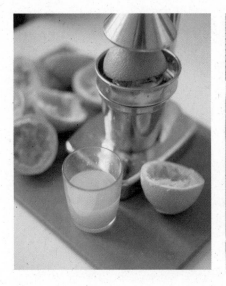
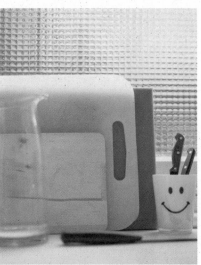

- It's got a glass jug – sturdy and easy to clean
- It's got a heavy base that the jug clicks into – again, sturdiness is key
- It has 2 different power settings, so it can chop on the low setting and blend on the high one.
- It has a pulse setting for gently integrating ingredients, e.g. it mixes in kiwi fruit without breaking down the seeds, which can be bitter
- It has power – 500 watts. Settle for less and your blender may pant and wheeze
- And the bits like going in the dishwasher

our squeezer

Not much we can really say about our citrus squeezer. It's one of those ones that looks a bit like a sombrero that you can buy in any decent kitchen supplies shop. We are guessing that you all know how it works – cut your orange in half along its equator, then ream out the juice on the pointy bit of the sombrero. Nice and simple. A bit like us really.

other stuff

You will also need a sharp knife, a chopping board and some fancy glasses to drink from, or you could sip directly from the jug if nobody's looking.

what do I do with this fruit?

juice it

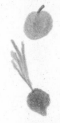

Apple – a juicing stalwart, used freely for its natural sweetness and ability to mix with virtually anything. Rich in beta-carotene and vitamin C, and great at helping the body to remove toxins.

Beetroot – a super juice, ruby-red and very sweet. Rich in iron, so very good for the blood, and also believed to detox the liver and help your guts work properly. Might make your wee pink too.

Broccoli – number one veg on the innocent hit parade. Its juice is a bit too strong on its own, but great when mixed. A nutrient powerhouse, stuffed full of antioxidants.

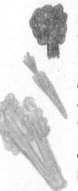

Carrot – arguably the finest, sweetest juice in all the land. Baby carrots are sweetest; big old ones can be a little bitter. The ultimate detoxifier, marvellous for a healthy liver and good for your guts.

Celery – its high water content makes it great for juicing. Contains potassium and folic acid, and is thought to aid digestion.

Melon – all melons can be juiced for their sweet nectar, but when ripe, you're better off blending them (see 'Blend it').

Pear – a fine mixer when juiced, naturally sweetening all smoothies. A great cleanser, so good for the intestines and for detoxifying your tired old body.

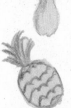

Pineapple – put them through your juicer for sweet nectar (when ripe they can also be blended whole for texture). Great for digestion and your guts.

Spinach – deep green spooky juice with a powerful taste. Rich in everything you need to stay healthy, including iron, potassium, beta-carotene, vitamin C, calcium. Get it into your juice now.

blend it

Avocado – blend them up to make very posh smoothies. Rich in both potassium and monounsaturated fat, which are both good sources of energy.

Banana – great for naturally thickening and sweetening your smoothies. And they contain all 8 of the amino acids that our bodies can't produce themselves. Clever.

Blackberry – a sweet, rich juice that's great with apples and pears. Rich in vitamin C, beta-carotene and also helps the immune system to function well.

Blackcurrant – sweet baubles of joy, super-rich in vitamin C. A great fruit to get into smoothies for kids.

Blueberry – great with any of its dark berry sisters or with yoghurt. Commonly believed to be the richest provider of antioxidants in the world of fruit and veg, pound for pound.

Cantaloupe melon – tons of vitamin A. In fact, a cupful of this juice will provide you with your recommended daily intake of the stuff.

Cherry – blend whole for sumptuous smoothies (remember to take the stones out). A good source of anthocyanins, natural pigments that are thought to help prevent cancer.

Coconut – if you're using tinned coconut milk, find one that doesn't use additives and stabilisers. Rich in zinc, potassium and a bit of vitamin C. Don't try blending whole coconuts or even the white flesh. Your blender won't like it.

Cranberry – very hard to find fresh so use frozen if necessary. Known for their great work in the area of the kidneys and the urinary tract.

Date – best when blended with yoghurt and honey. And a very fine place to find a bit of calcium and iron for better blood and bones.

Kiwi – a good place to get your vitamin C, which should help keep your immune system working well. Don't over-blend, or you'll crush the seeds and your drink will taste peppery.

Lychee – yet another good source of vitamin C and very posh to boot. A lady's love of lychees once started a war in China, but we haven't got time to go into that now.

Mango – these beauties are packed with beta-carotene, which helps to maintain healthy eyesight and glowing skin.

Nectarine – a fine provider of beta-carotene, magnesium and folic acid, the last being important for pregnant women.

Passion fruit – surprisingly rich in vitamin A, as well as being a good source of vitamin C, iron and potassium. Tough stuff for one so delicately named.

Peach – pretty much like nectarines, except hairier.

Pineapple – these spiky chaps contain bromelain, an enzyme that aids the digestive process. Pineapples are also a good source of manganese, which boosts energy production.

Prune – let's not beat about the bush. We all know what they're good for. Off you go with the newspaper.

Raspberry – when they're in season, make sure they're in your smoothies. An expert at cleansing your guts and helping out with your waterworks as well.

Strawberry – blend whole for deep red smoothies. Contain a multitude of nutrients, including potassium, which provides natural energy.

Watermelon — great for rehydration and getting your waterworks to function nicely. Also a good source of vitamin C and the antioxidant lycopene.

squeeze it

 Lemon – naturally sharp and great at giving spark to a smoothie or juice. Lots of vitamin C and very cleansing – great detox juice.

 Lime – a bit like lemons but smaller and greener.

 Orange – a smoothie staple, providing sweetness and tang. Great source of vitamin C, but we didn't really need to tell you that, did we?

the golden rules of juicing

We've been making smoothies and juices for years. So we thought we'd pass on some of our favourite miscellaneous didn't-fit-anywhere-else tips before we got to the recipes. In no particular order, here are the golden rules of juicing:

Trust your senses. Fruit and veg vary in size, taste and quality during the year, as befits something wholly natural. So don't be scared to alter the amounts that you use in order to make your drink taste the best. Cut loose. Live on the edge.

Stay clean. Always always wash your fruit and veg before you blend or juice it. It's a no-brainer really. Who knows where it's been?

Ignore us. Don't stick to the recipe – make up your own stuff. That's how we came up with these recipes. And if you come up with any winners, send them in and we'll stick them in the next book. Your mum will be so proud.

Be runny. The best smoothies are made by starting off with the runny stuff. For example, if you were making an apple and banana drink, juice your apples with a juicer first, then pour the apple juice into the blender. Add the banana bit by bit and blend until you get the desired consistency.

Don't bother with boosters. Nature provides so much amazing stuff that you don't need to add weird powders and potions. Stick to fruit and veg, for they will serve you well.

Keep your carrots cold. A fairly specific one – warm carrot juice isn't great, so pop your carrots into the fridge for a while before you juice them.

Cheat with apples. Lots of our recipes use an apple juice base. If you can't be bothered to juice apples every time, you can always sub them with some nice fresh pressed apple juice from a carton or bottle.

Switch it off. Sometimes you might get a bit of fruit stuck in the bottom of your nice juicer or blender. The temptation is to try to free it with your fingers – bad call, especially if you haven't unplugged it first. We'd like you to keep your fingers.

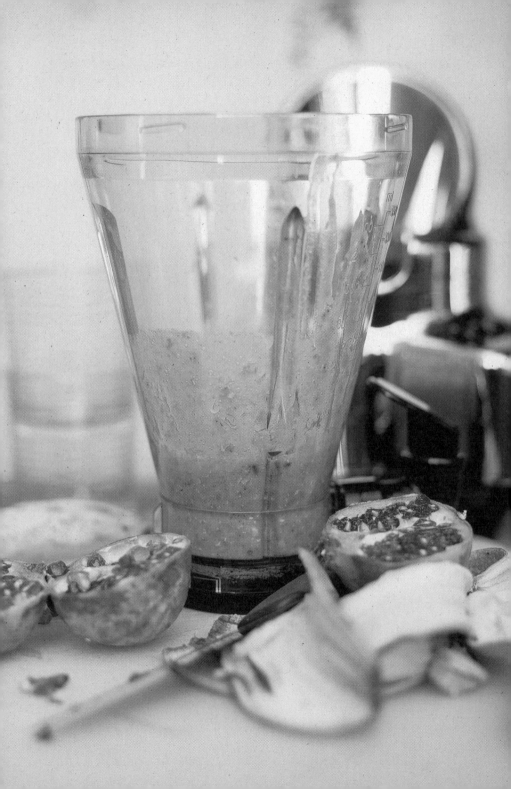

smoothies

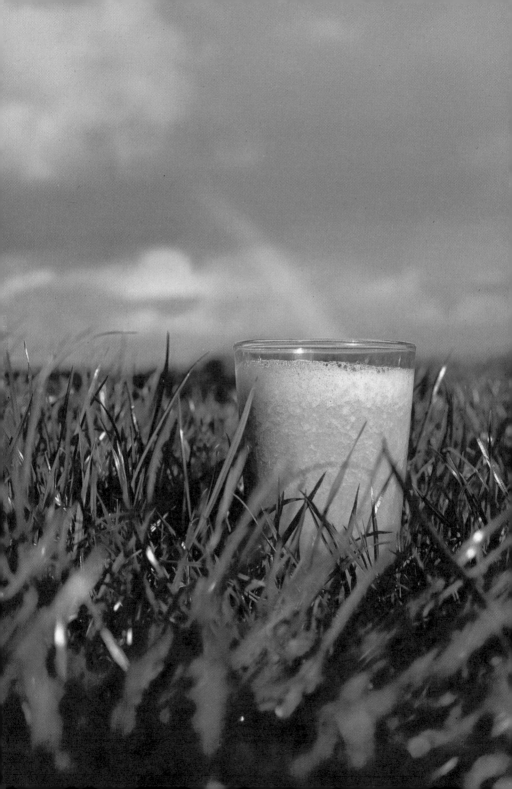

strawberry and banana

This is where it all began. An old classic, a family favourite, a timeless recipe from an era when things seemed a little more, erm, innocent. Anyway, this is the exact same recipe you'll find in our bottles, so it should taste good.

what you need
2½ apples
7 strawberries
½ an orange
½ a banana

what to do
Cut the apple into wedges and put them through the juicer. Squeeze half an orange. Pour both apple juice and orange juice into the blender. Add the strawberries and banana and blend away. 1 generous serving.

Make sure your fruit is clean by rinsing it under the tap before you start. Dirty fruit ain't much fun.

mango and passion fruit

Glenn Medeiros. Engelbert Humperdinck. Alphonso mangoes. These are some of our favourite smooth things. Especially the last one. In fact, we reckon that the Alphonso's velvety texture and smooth fragrant taste is so fine that it'll have you singing a power ballad in no time at all.

what you need
½ a juicy mango
½ a banana
2½ apples
1 wrinkly passion fruit
½ an orange

what to do
Peel the mango and slice it into the blender. Pop the banana into the blender as well. Cut the apple into wedges and put them through the juicer. Strain the juice from the passion fruit (don't add the seeds) into the blender, using a sieve. Add the apple juice and the juice of half an orange to the blender and whizz everything until smooth. Pour over ice and sip. 1 generous serving.

Peel off the banana's stringy bits before blending. They taste bitter, and you don't really want that.

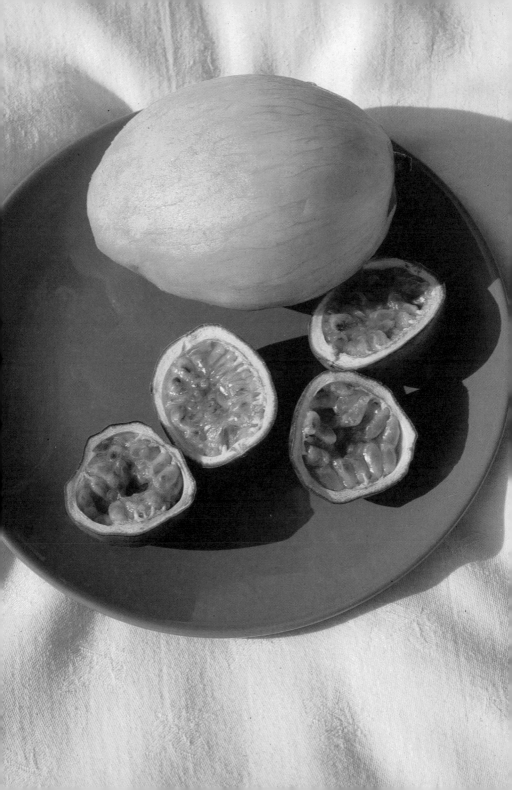

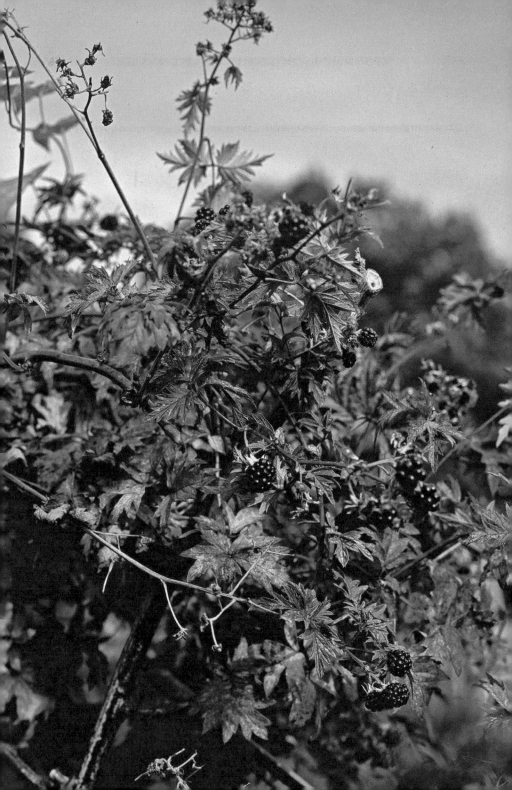

blackberry and blueberry

This recipe is sublime. But it's even more sublime if you go down to the woods and find some wild blueberries, seeing as they taste a little bit better than the farmed ones. Go on. Off you pop. Take your tent and your rifle and hunt them down. Stay downwind of them so they don't catch your scent.

what you need
2½ apples
½ a banana
1 punnet of blueberries
1 punnet of blackberries
½ an orange

what to do
Cut the apple into wedges, put them through the juicer and pour the juice into a blender. Add the berries and half a peeled banana to the blender with a dash of freshly squeezed OJ. Blitz until you get the desired consistency. 1 generous serving.

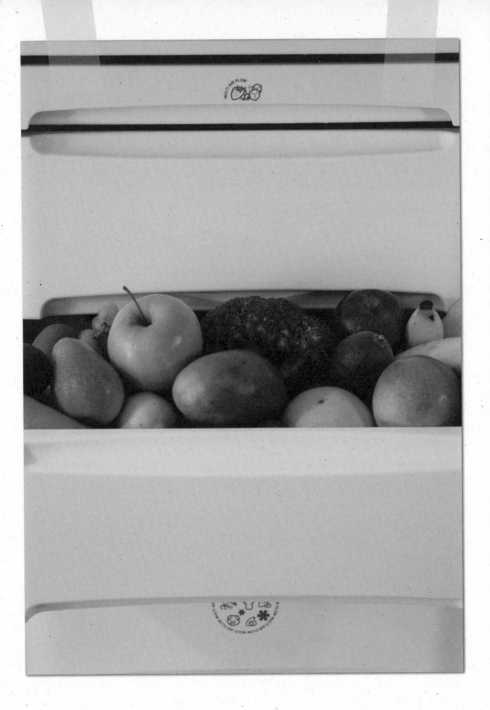

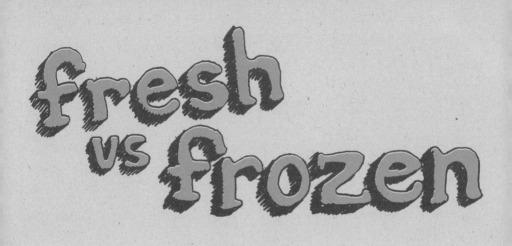

fresh vs frozen

Freezers are cold places, but don't let this put you off. Underneath all that frostiness is something that's actually quite useful. You see, freezers keep stuff fresh for longer. Fact: freezing food doesn't sterilise it or make it nutritionally worthless. All it does is slow down the growth of the microorganisms that make food go off.

So, freezing is your friend. In fact, lots of people prefer to make smoothies with frozen ingredients. You can get lots of fruit, especially berries, already frozen. Or you can buy your weekly dose of fruit and veg, prep it and freeze it, so that it's sitting there waiting to be made into smoothies in the morning, when clearly the last thing you want to do is chop up lots of fruit and veg.

Please note – there is some boring stuff to know about freezing fruit and veg. Prep fruit as if you were about to use it, so peel it, chop it, take the stones out and pop it in a freezer bag before freezing. Veg is a bit more of a pain – wash, trim and chop it as normal, and if it's a root veggie, blanch it for a couple of minutes, chill it in ice cold water for another couple of minutes, pat it dry and freeze in a bag or airtight plastic container.

Told you it was boring.

avocado and pear

Debbie sent us this recipe. She says that she's bored of inventing smoothies at home and hopes that someone will write a decent smoothie recipe book to give her some new ideas. Ahem.

what you need
3 pears
½ a lemon
2 oranges
1 avocado

what to do
Cut the pear into wedges, put them through the juicer and pour the juice into the blender. Squeeze the juice from the lemon and oranges and add to the blender. Cut the avocado in half, remove the stone, scoop out the flesh and add to the blender. Whizz until everything is blended together. 2 servings.

Debbie is a girl's name, whereas something like Alex can be used for both sexes.

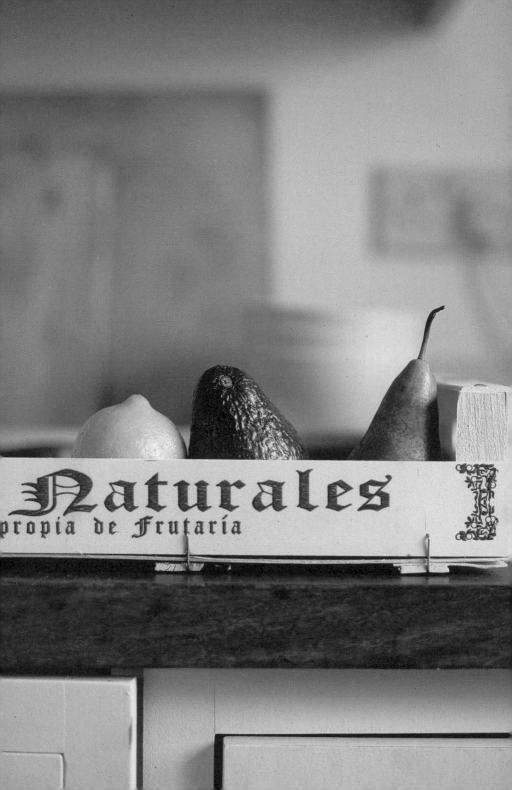

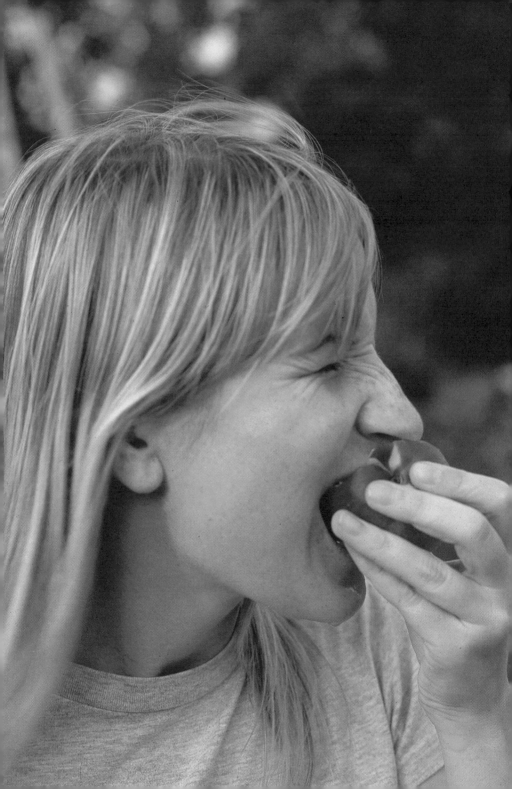

strawberry and nectarine

Biting into a nectarine and allowing the juice to run down your chin is a social faux pas, right up there with licking your knife in a posh restaurant or calling the Queen 'mate' when you bump into her at the races. Avoid such embarrassing situations by popping your nectarines into smoothies such as this one, and leave those ill-mannered days behind you.

what you need
2 apples
1 ½ nectarines
6 strawberries

what to do
Cut the apples into wedges and put them through the juicer. Cut the nectarine into chunks, discarding the stone. Roughly chop the strawberries. Chuck everything (apple juice, strawbs and nectarines) into the blender and do the blending. 2 servings.

Use peaches if you can't find nectarines.
Nothing wrong with a bit of fuzz in your drink.

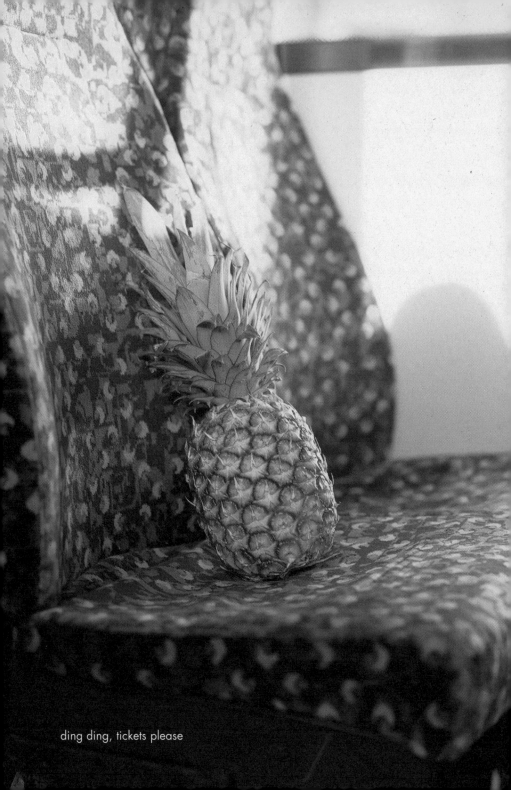

ding ding, tickets please

orange, banana and pineapple

All of these ingredients were meant to be together, like star-crossed lovers on a moonlit night who ran out of the disco and into each other's arms, got the bus home together, drank coffee, got married three months' later and now have a little baby called Jason.

what you need
1 succulent pineapple
1 orange
1 banana
A wedge of lime

what to do
Peel and core the pineapple. Put half of the pineapple through the juicer. Cut the other half into chunks and put them into the blender. Squeeze the juice from one orange and add it, the pineapple juice and the peeled banana to the blender. Add a squeeze of lime juice. Blend until smooth. 2 generous servings.

Add a dollop of natural yoghurt if there's some in the fridge. Please don't use mayonnaise as a substitute.

How to clean your juicer*

You may have already seen our tips on what kind of kit to buy to make all of these drinks. There's loads of good equipment out there, and most of it is pretty easy to clean and look after.

However, there is only so much a person can take. After lots of juicing and blending, a certain type of rage can build up – the sort that comes from thinking 'It's dirty and I can't be bothered to clean it again.'

So here is a patented innocent stress-buster. We call it 'Cleaning Your Juicer With a Hammer'.

*with a hammer

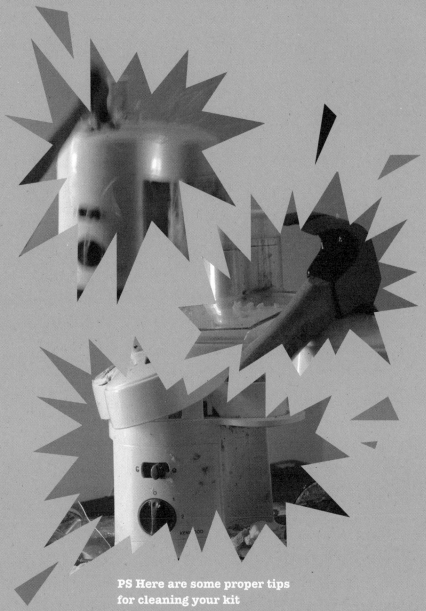

**PS Here are some proper tips
for cleaning your kit**

1. Check that the parts are dishwasherable before
   you purchase.
2. Get a juicer with a big removable waste container.
3. After you've juiced, put a lemon through your juicer.
   It'll naturally clean and freshen the gizmo.
4. Get your mum to come round and clean it.

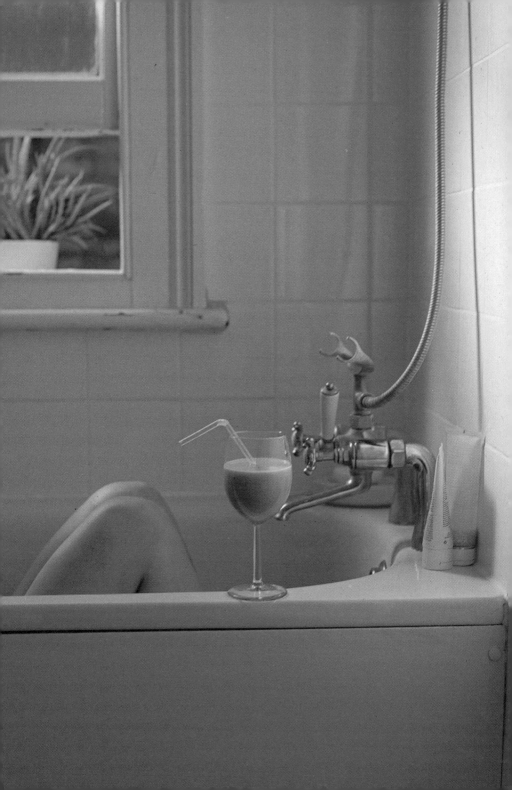

papaya, lime and coconut

More tropical than two weeks in the Maldives, this smoothie is best drunk when in the holiday mood. So nip down to B&Q, buy a few bags of sand, chuck a load of salt in your bath and create your own beach, right there in the bathroom. For added authenticity, ask the neighbours to pop round every 15 minutes with a few wooden elephants in case you feel like buying one.

what you need
1 medium-sized papaya
½ a pineapple
½ a lime
½ a banana
2 dessertspoons of coconut cream

what to do
Cut the papaya open and remove the seeds. Slice the flesh (without skin) into the blender. Peel the pineapple, chop it into bits and juice it. Add the pineapple juice, banana, coconut cream and lime juice and zest to the blender. Whizz it all until you get something nice and smooth. 1 generous serving.

Some say papaya, some say paw paw. But they're one and the same.

cantaloupe and peach

'Cantaloupe & Peach' sound a bit like a French pop act, but sadly it's just another smoothie recipe, albeit a very tasty one. And a very healthy one too. You see, melon juice is a great rehydrator, so may we suggest that you partake of this one at the end of a hot day, or perhaps after a heavy night down the Dog and Clarinet?

what you need
½ an apple (or 25ml of fresh apple juice if you're feeling lazy)
¼ of a cantaloupe melon
2 peaches
1 orange
½ a banana
1 wedge of lemon

what to do
Cut the apple into wedges, put them through the juicer and pour the juice into the blender. Chop the melon flesh into chunks and add to the blender, along with the chopped-up peaches (stones removed). Squeeze the juice from your orange. Put everything except the lemon into the blender and whizz. Finish off by stirring in a squeeze of lemon juice. 2 servings.

We are not melon fascists. If you want to use watermelon or honeydew, that's what you should do.

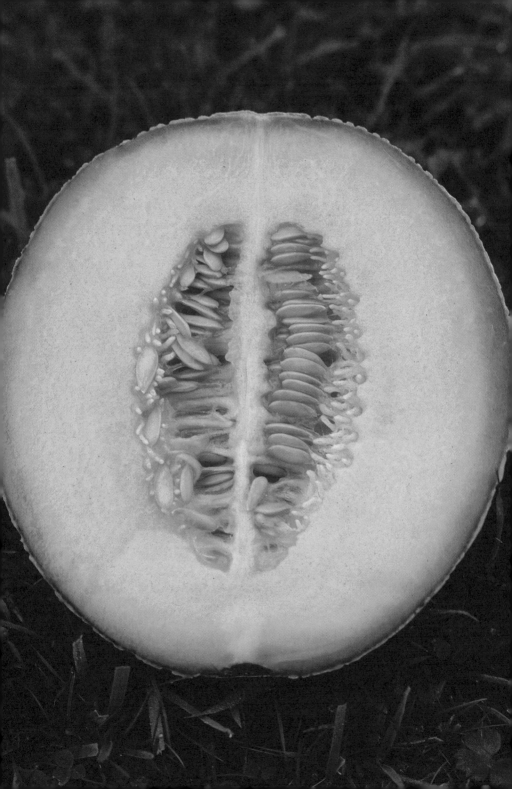

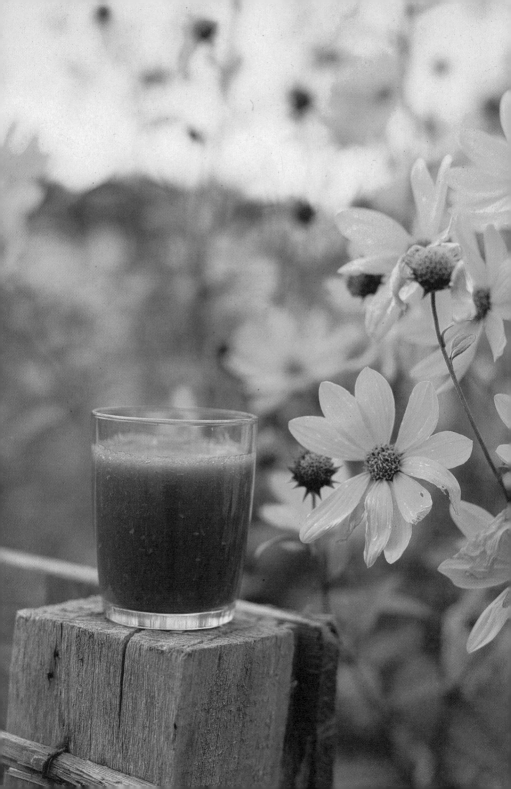

summer in a glass

You don't know when you've got it good, I tell you. When I was a lad, we couldn't get summer in a glass, oh no. Couldn't even get it in a brown paper bag. Had to sit outside in a cardboard box all winter and spring, waiting for summer to come along, with only a bottle of stout to see us through.

what you need
¼ of a cantaloupe melon
A handful of cherries
A large sprig of blackcurrants
A small punnet of raspberries
2 apples

what to do
Remove and discard the rind and the seeds of the melon. Chop the melon into chunks. Halve the cherries and remove the stones. Add the melon, cherries, blackcurrants and raspberries to the blender. Cut the apples into wedges, put them through the juicer and pour the juice into the blender. Whizz everything together until blended. 2 servings.

cherries, raspberries and blackcurrants all contain anthocyanins, powerful antioxidants that do battle with any filthy toxins that may be in your body.

the while-u-wait workout

You're busy. Time is short. But you need to get fit somehow.
So here are some exercises to keep you trim while you're juicing.

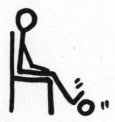

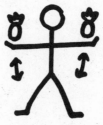

sole food

push pineapple

Take a couple of coconuts, sit on a chair, place them on the floor under your feet and roll them around vigorously for a couple of minutes. The massaging effect will soothe your tired toes and the coarse coconut shell is nature's answer to the £79 pedicure. NB Wash your feet first.

What's more, you don't have to shake the tree. Just take two pineapples (or other heavy fruit), hold one in each hand down by your side and then lift, in a motion that is similar to a bird flapping its wings. Except don't flap – hold for 10 seconds when your arms reach the horizontal position, and then lower slowly. Repeat 10 times.

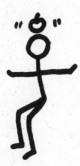

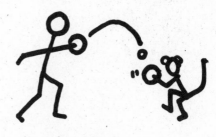

william tell

Take a shiny apple, balance it on top of your head and see if you can make it round the kitchen table without it falling off your head. This one's all about poise and balance – great for your spine and your trunk.

monkey tennis

Find a monkey and play tennis with it. You could use an orange as the ball and some kitchen plates as racquets. Winner gets a banana.

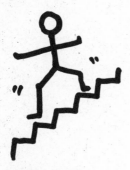

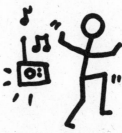

the wooden hill

After you've chopped up all of your ingredients, go and do five minutes on the stairs – run up and down them, going from side to side just like in those old movies with Fred Astaire. The fancier your footwork, the more good you'll be doing the muscles in your legs and bum, and the more out of breath you get, the better it is for your heart.

fly moves

Dancing is great. Before you turn on your blender, turn on the radio, find something with a rhythm to your liking and cut loose. Frug, twist, jive, and body rock your way to aerobic fitness for a solid five minutes – at the end of it you should be out of breath, which means that it's doing your heart some good.
PS You might want to pull the curtains, just in case the neighbours are looking in.

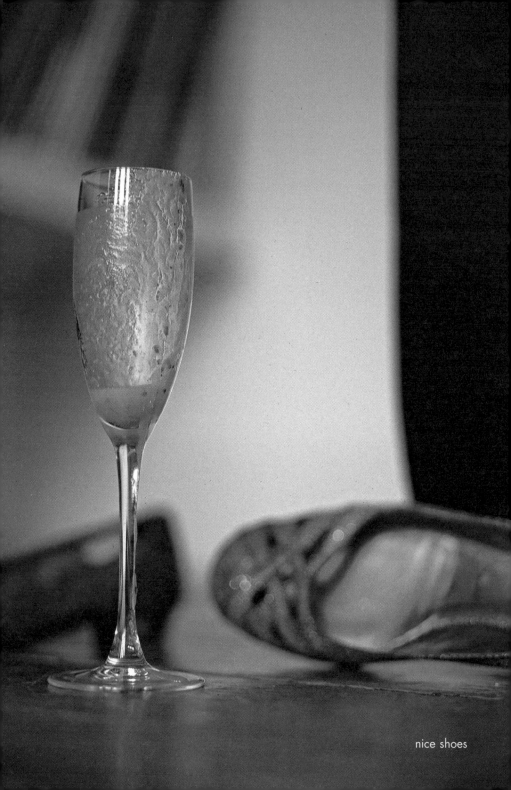

nice shoes

honeyed pears and ginger

Honeyed pears are a bit posh. In fact, they sound like something that should be on the menu down at Le Trop Cher. So please, put on your best frock, do your hair, get the best china out and give this one a go. You may find that wearing a monocle and talking about polo ponies really tops off the whole posh thing, but don't feel that you have to go overboard on our account.

what you need
1 soft juicy pear
Some honey
A thumbnail of fresh ginger
2 oranges

what to do
Switch your grill on. Cut the pear in half. Take out the core and stalk and put the halves on a baking tray (flesh side up). Brush with honey and grill for 5–10 minutes – until the flesh is slightly soft and the honey caramelises. Peel and finely chop the ginger and chuck it in the blender with the orange juice. Add the honeyed pears and blend. 1 serving.

We'd advise using Comice pears if you can find some. They're very aromatic. As for honey, we used orange blossom honey. Complements the ginger perfectly. Ooh la la.

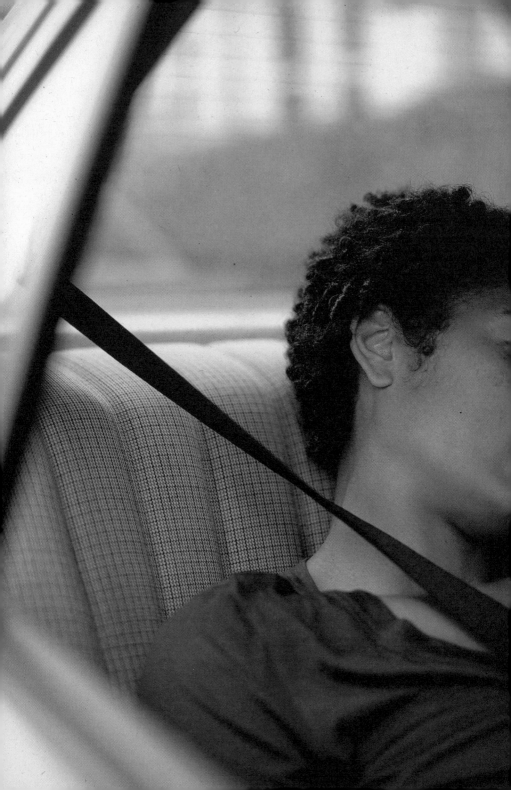

pineapple, blueberry and ginger

Ginger has been an important part of Chinese medicine for centuries. It's also a good name for a cat. But we digress. Today we want to tell you about how ginger can help you when you're feeling bad during a long car journey. Next time you're turning green in the back seat, try peeling a small piece of ginger and chewing it. It should make for a more pleasant trip and you won't need to wear those weird wristbands either. Safe journey.

what you need
½ an orange
½ a pineapple
½ a banana
2 handfuls of blueberries
A nice bit of fresh ginger

what to do
Squeeze the juice from the orange. Remove the skin from the pineapple, chop into chunks and put them through the juicer. Peel and chop the banana and pop it in the blender with the blueberries, orange and pineapple juice. Peel and finely grate a nice chunk (1–2cm) of ginger into the blender. Whizz and serve. 1 generous serving.

This recipe was made in detox heaven, seeing as it contains three of the most detox-friendly ingredients ever. Blueberries are packed with antioxidants, ginger is a fantastic natural cleanser and pineapple contains bromelain, which aids digestion. Nice.

chinese pear and star anise

The Chinese pears that we used in this recipe are the variety known as Tientsin. They stay crisp when other pears go soft, and they give a lot of juice to boot. If you can't find any in the shops, you could substitute a very crisp apple to go in their place, although this would obviously change the flavour a fair bit. And it wouldn't be very Chinese.

what you need
3 crunchy Chinese pears
1 orange
1 banana
A large pinch of finely ground star anise
A wedge of lemon

what to do
Cut the pears into wedges, put them through the juicer and pour the juice into the blender. Freshly squeeze the orange and add the juice to the blender. Chop up the banana and pop that in the blender too. Finally, add the finely ground star anise to the blender with a squeeze of lemon juice. Pulse until you get to smoothie heaven. 2 servings.

This drink oxidises (goes brown) quite quickly. Please knock it back pronto.

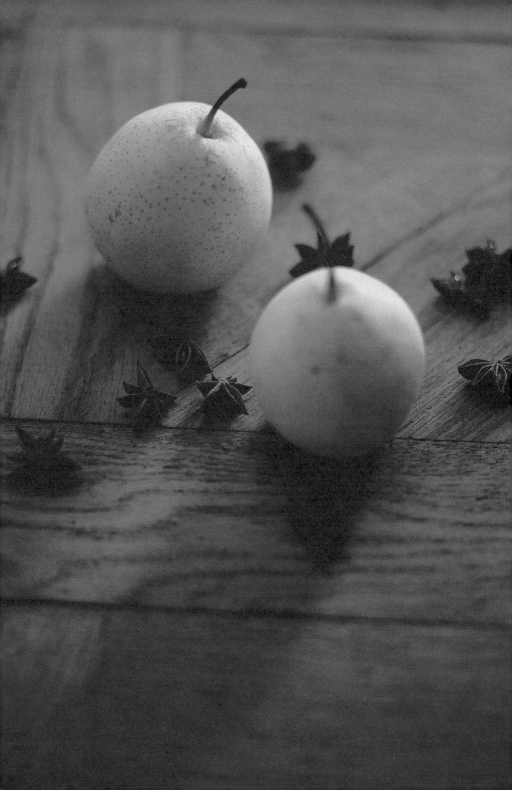

a toast to absent friends

When it comes to inventing smoothies, we've tried most things. But some ingredients just don't work. Some combinations taste like bad medicine. Allow us to take you on a tour of the stuff that didn't make it.

tofu

We had good intentions. Tofu makes us feel worthy. But in a drink, it's just tof-ugly.

onion juice

Wrong in so many ways. Looks like yellow milk, tastes like onion juice. Drink it and you will lose all of your friends.

clam juice

We once tested this out on Will, our American friend. His face went funny. Funny peculiar.

oranges and almonds

We like oranges and we like almonds. But when they're together, something bad happens, like the opposite of when Torvill met Dean.

cauliflower juice

You may be great with cheese, but never, ever come near my juicer again.
Do you hear me?
Take a walk, sunbeam.
Stick to the cheese.

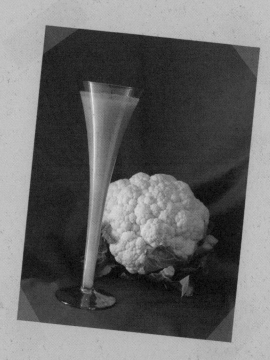

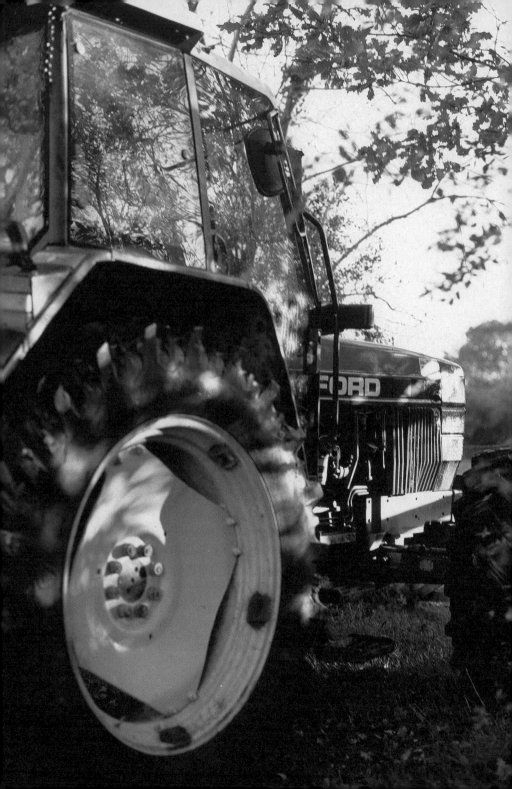

blackcurrant and lychee

Our favourite blackcurrants come from a farm in Herefordshire, run by a nice chap called Edward. The last time we went to visit, we had a go on his tractor. Brilliant.

what you need
1 apple
1 orange
6 lychees
½ a banana
16 blackcurrants (precision is everything)

what to do
Cut the apple into wedges and put them through the juicer. Squeeze the orange and put both apple and orange juice in the blender. Peel and stone the lychees and peel and chop the banana. Pop everything into the blender, whizz and serve. 2 servings.

feeling lucky? Stick a scoop of elderflower or lemon sorbet on top for a smoothie float.

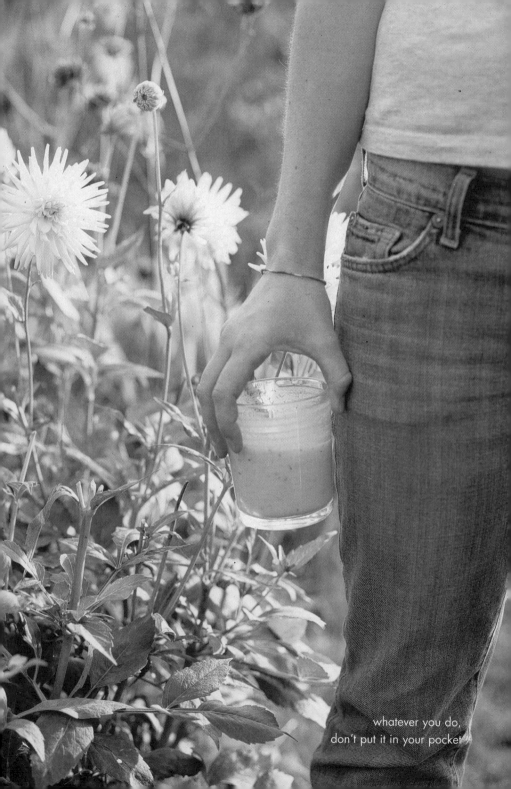

whatever you do,
don't put it in your pocket

pineapple, lychees, peach and lemongrass

This recipe was sent to us by an innocent drinker called Natasha. For six months of the year she lives in Hong Kong (all right for some) and she says that this one is for 'the days that it's grim outside and you dream of an exotic island where the sun always shines'. Hear! hear!

what you need
½ a pineapple
10 lychees
½ a banana
1 peach
100ml of coconut milk
A pinch of lemongrass

what to do
Remove the skin from the pineapple and cut it into chunks. Put these through the juicer and pour the juice into the blender. Peel and stone the lychees and add the flesh to the blender. Halve the peach, remove the stone and slice into the blender. Chuck the banana in and whizz everything together. Finely chop about a centimetre of lemongrass, discarding the tough outer leaves. Add the coconut milk and a pinch of the chopped lemongrass to the blender. Pulse the blender 4 times and drink. 2 servings.

pomegranate and blueberry

When you're looking for a recipe to lift you out of a hole, have a go with this little aluminium ladder of a smoothie. Pomegranates and blueberries are amazing sources of antioxidants, which help to keep your immune system strong and will fight rogue cells called free radicals, which are intent on doing you harm. The perfect recipe for the times when your mind and body are conspiring against you.

what you need
1 apple
1 pomegranate
½ a punnet of blueberries
½ a banana
1 orange

what to do
Cut the apple into wedges, put them through the juicer and pour the juice into the blender. Squeeze the orange and pour the juice into the blender too. Cut the pomegranate into quarters. Fold back the skin of each quarter and remove the seeds. Put them through the juicer then add this juice to the blender along with the blueberries and half a banana. Whizz until smooth. 1 serving.

Pomegranates are a symbol of fertility.
Go forth and get busy

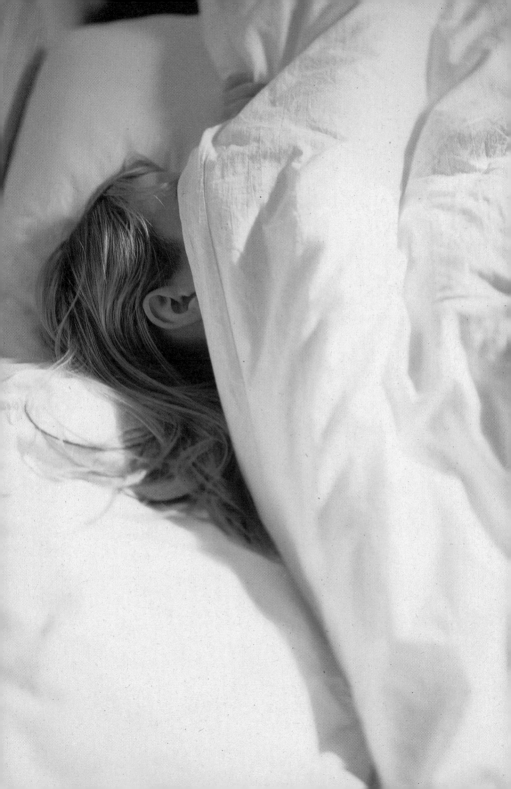

thickies

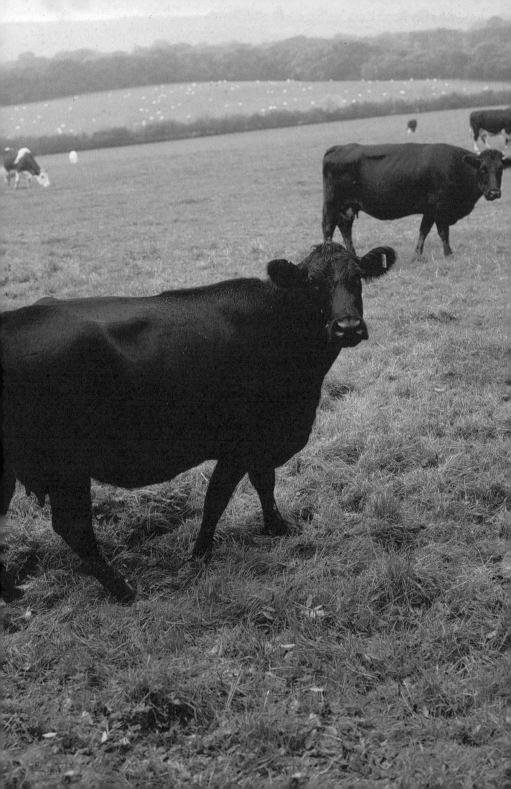

yoghurt, vanilla bean and honey

They say that you shouldn't have favourites. Try telling that to a bookmaker. Anyway, we have favourites and we're not embarrassed to say that this is one of them. It's the first thickie we ever made and it still seems to be our most popular recipe if the weird love noises that people make after taking their first mouthful are anything to go by.

what you need
2 large apples
1 teaspoon of honey
4 tablespoons of bio-yoghurt
¼ of a vanilla pod

what to do
Cut the apples into wedges and put through the juicer. Put the apple juice, honey and yoghurt into the blender. Scrape the seeds from the vanilla pod into the blender and pulse twice. 1 generous serving.

Don't overblend this one, as the yoghurt will get too thin. And use acacia honey if you can find some. Tastes magic.

blackberry and lavender

The scent of lavender reminds us of being in Grandma's garden, as the summer light dwindles and a cool breeze blows another day to a close. But there's still time for you to do your chores, you lazy so and so. Mow the lawn, do the weeding and polish the gnomes – if you're lucky you might get 50p for an ice cream.

what you need
2 apples
8 plump blackberries
3 teaspoons of lavender honey
200g of natural bio-yoghurt
Lavender flowers to decorate, if you're feeling fancy

what to do
Cut the apple into wedges, put them through the juicer and pour the juice into the blender. Add the blackberries and honey to the blender and blend until mixed. Add the yoghurt and pulse twice. 2 servings.

We used lavender honey from Paynes Southdown Bee Farms Ltd. www.paynes-beefarm.com

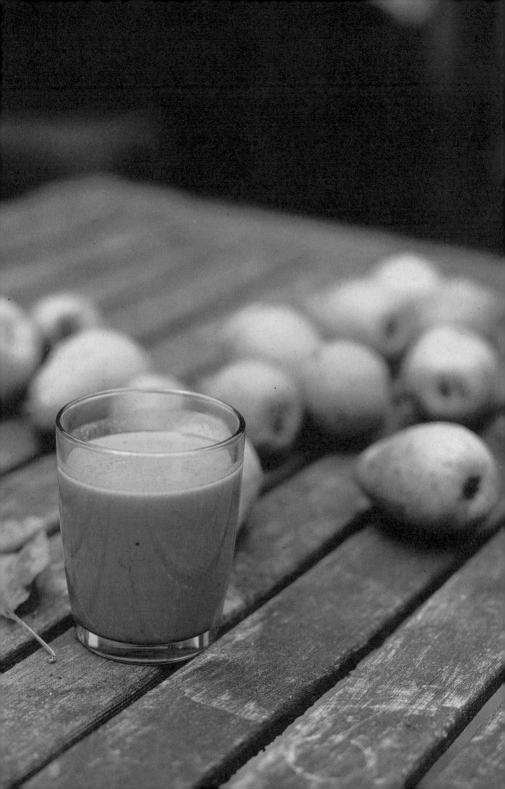

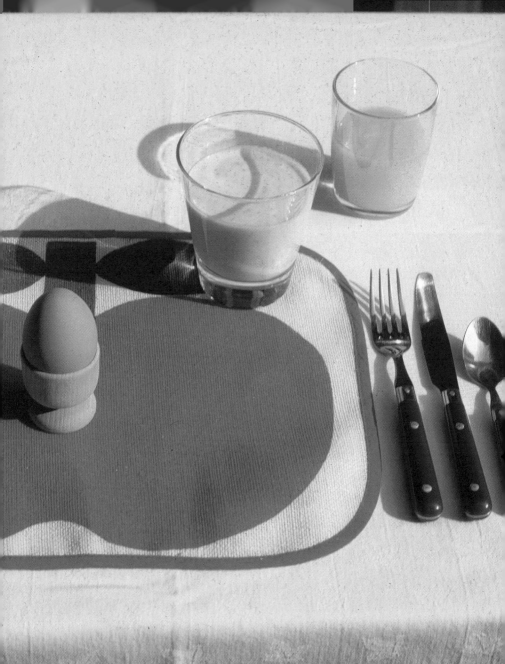

where are the soldiers? this is a disgrace

banana, oats
and medjool dates

What is it they say? Breakfast like a CEO, lunch like a middle manager and have your dinner whilst watching *Holby City* on the mini-telly in the night-watchman's cabin. Something like that. Anyway, breakfast is important and we reckon that this is the best breakfast drink on Earth. It's got oats for all of that slow release low GI energy you've been reading about. And bananas, honey and dates, which aren't too shabby in the energy department either. Just watch yourself go.

what you need
2 apples
½ a banana
2 teaspoons of acacia honey
3 medjool dates
200g of natural yoghurt
20g of oats

what to do
Cut the apple into wedges, put them through the juicer and pour into the blender. Add the banana, honey and dates to the blender. Whizz until nice and smooth. Add the yoghurt and oats and pulse 4 times. 2 servings.

If yoghurt doesn't agree with you, use 200ml of soya milk instead. And check the pack — soya milk from the bean is best, rather than the stuff made from isolates, whatever they are.

the people behind the drinks

It's fair to say that without these people, this book wouldn't exist. Our drinks wouldn't exist. Our company wouldn't exist. You may think we're being melodramatic, but we're not, because these are the people who invent our recipes, who check our drinks every day to make sure they taste amazing, who know everything there is to know about making smoothies. Ladies and gentlemen, we give you our ladies of the kitchen.

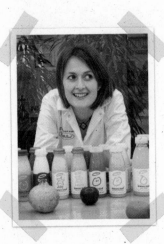

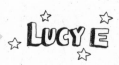 LUCY E

The boss. Has the rest of the team in her steely grip.

 Nikki

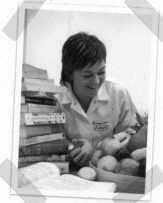

The brains of the operation. Nothing gets past her.

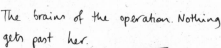

LUCY T

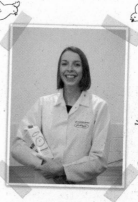

The caring face of the kitchen.
She's from Wales.

Eleanor

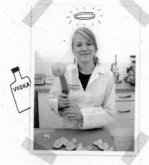

The very picture of innocence. But looks can
be deceiving.

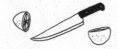

Amy

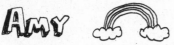

Our very own market trader. Knows everything
there is to know about our ingredients.

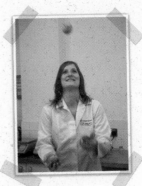

SARAH

The new kid. Sassy, street smart and some
other stuff that begins with 's'!

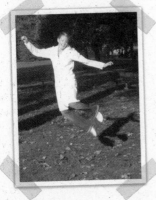
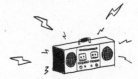

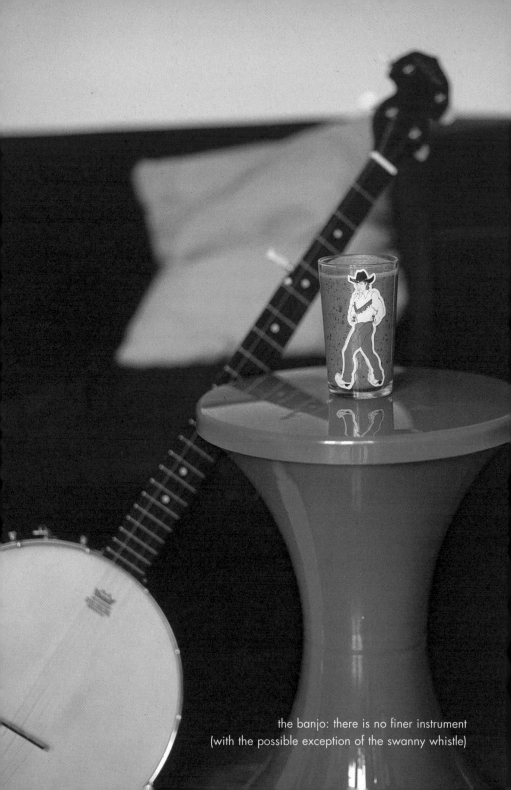

the banjo: there is no finer instrument
(with the possible exception of the swanny whistle)

blueberry, maple syrup and oats

Gosh darn it ma'am, this sure is the tastiest little breakfast drink I ever did see, yessirree. (That was our impression of somebody from the United States enjoying this fine breakfast thickie. We hope you enjoyed it.)

what you need
½ an apple (or 25ml of fresh apple juice if you're feeling lazy)
A punnet of blueberries
2 dessertspoons of maple syrup
250ml of bio-yoghurt
A small handful of oats
Pecan nuts to serve

what to do
Cut the apple into wedges and put them through the juicer. Add the apple juice, blueberries and the maple syrup to the blender and whizz until smooth. Add the yoghurt and oats and pulse twice. Serve sprinkled with chopped pecan nuts. 1 generous serving.

Don't use maple "flavoured" syrup if possible - the real maple stuff's the best.

mango, coconut and lemongrass

If this thickie was a country, it would have to be Thailand. It's got all of the essential ingredients. All we need now is a couple of tuk-tuks and perhaps an elephant. Feel free to add your own.

what you need
2 large apples
1 medium-sized mango
4 tablespoons of coconut milk
A pinch of chopped lemongrass
4 tablespoons of bio-yoghurt
1 teaspoon of honey

what to do
Cut the apples into wedges, put them through the juicer and pour the juice into the blender. Peel the mango, remove the stone and cut the flesh into chunks. Add them to the blender. Discard the tough outer leaves of the lemongrass, take a centimetre-long piece and chop finely. Add the chopped lemongrass to the blender and whizz. Then add the coconut milk, yoghurt and honey and give everything a final pulse or two. 2 servings.

Try to use coconut milk without added stabilisers or gums, because stabilisers and gums are rubbish.

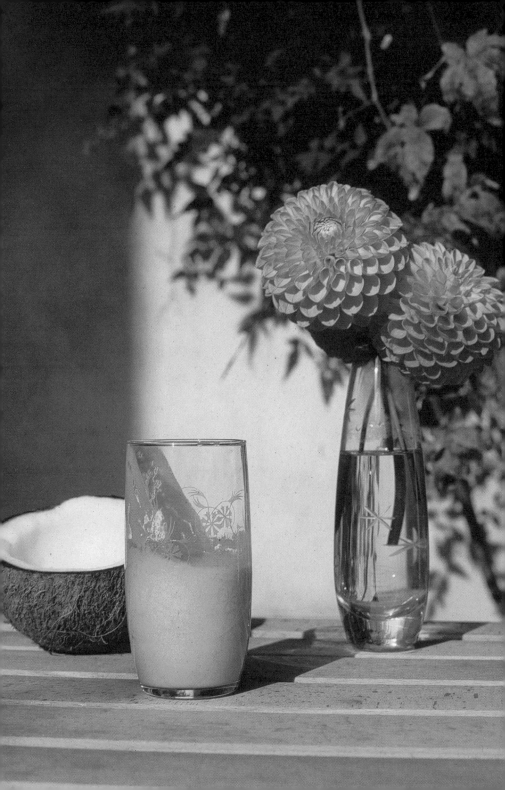

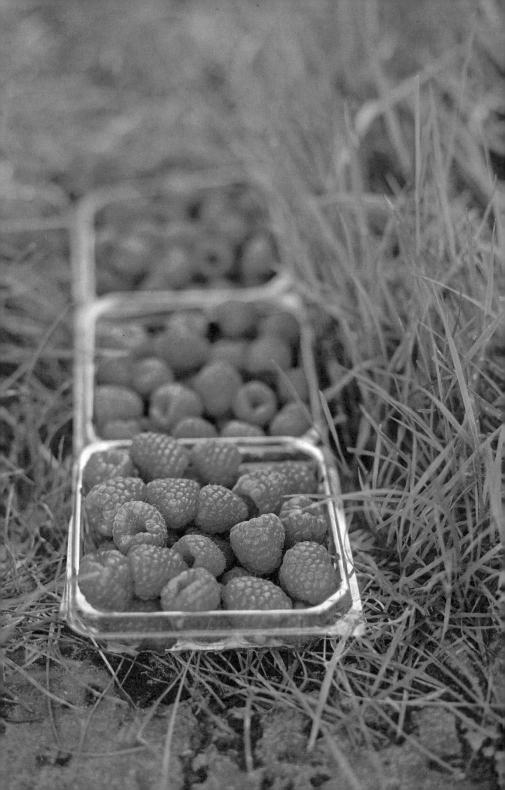

peach melba

The phrase 'do a Melba' means to return from retirement, or to make several farewell appearances (a bit like Status Quo). It comes from the name of the Australian operatic soprano Dame Nellie Melba, who loved nothing better than a good comeback show. Of course, this fact has got nothing to do with the recipe, but we thought it might help out if you're stuck for something to say at a forthcoming social engagement.

what you need
2 apples
2 juicy peaches
A punnet of raspberries
1 teaspoon of honey
200ml of natural bio-yoghurt

what to do
Cut the apples into wedges and put them through the juicer. Stone, then slice the peaches into the blender, then blend together with the raspberries, apple juice and honey until smooth. Add the yoghurt and pulse twice. 2 servings.

You only get one life. No receipt, no proof of purchase. You can't take it back to the shops if you're bored.

Hence the fact that you should appreciate what you've got. Find a job you love, find some people you love, visit your grandparents and get to the seaside as often as possible.

Eat well and eat cake. Go running, go jumping. Get your five a day.

Feed the cat. Fix your bike.
Have a baby and smoke a cigar.

Camp in the woods, bake some
bread and buy a trampoline.

Not necessarily in that order.

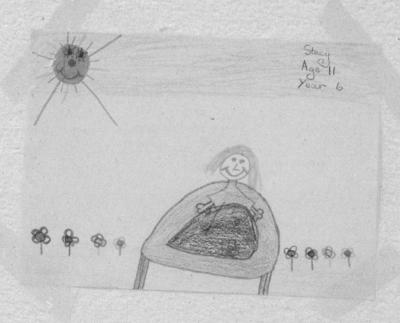

Stacy
Age 11
Year 6

breakfast on the beach

This recipe was sent in by Guni, who has been emailing us for years now, suggesting things and having a bit of a chat. We thought we'd thank her for her time by printing one of her favourite recipes. We love you, Guni.

what you need
1 orange
½ a pineapple
1 banana
75ml of skimmed milk
100ml of coconut milk
A sprinkling of oats

what to do
Squeeze the orange. Remove the skin and core from the pineapple and chop the flesh into chunks. Whizz everything, except the oats, in the blender until nice and smooth. Stir the oats into the drink and serve. 2 servings.

Oats are filled with cholesterol-reducing soluble fibre. So, erm, get your oats.

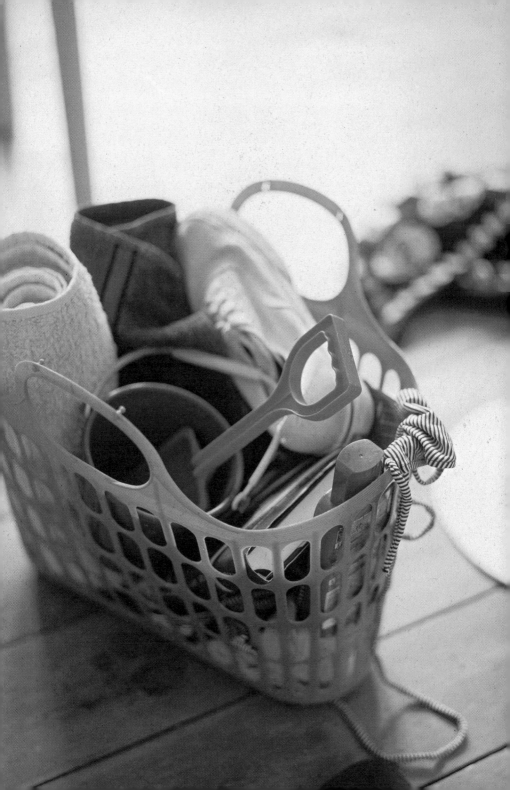

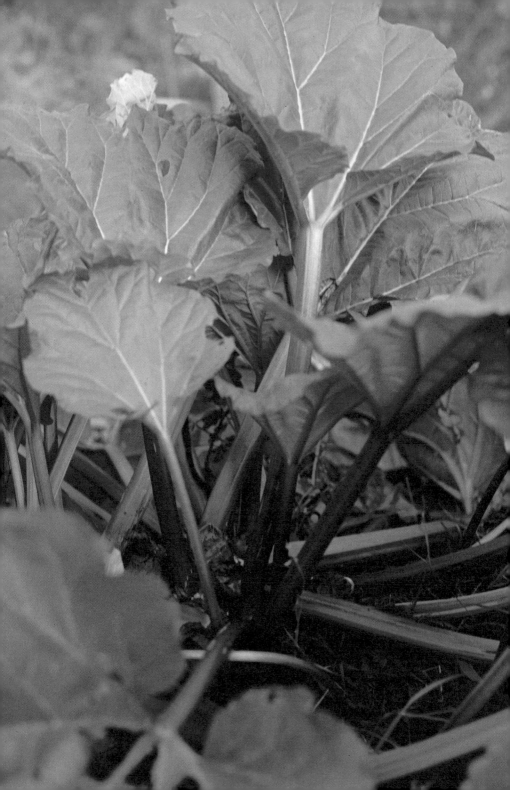

strawberry and rhubarb

Rhubarb rhubarb. And some strawberries, yoghurt, apples and honey.

what you need
1 apple
1 stick of rhubarb
6 strawberries
4 tablespoons of bio-yoghurt
1 teaspoon of honey

what to do
Cut the apple into wedges and put them through the juicer. Cut the rhubarb stick into chunks and place them in a saucepan with the apple juice. Cover and stew over a gentle heat for five or six minutes until the rhubarb is soft. When the rhubarb and apple are cool, pour them into the blender with the roughly chopped strawberries, yoghurt and honey and blend together. 2 servings.

Rhubarb is actually a vegetable and is a good source of vitamins A and C, as well as potassium and fibre.

rainbows are prettier than prunes, hence the picture

prune and nutmeg

So you think you're a tough guy? You think you've got what it takes to get to the top in this dog-eat-dog world? Well, prove it. Drink this tough guy drink. Down in one. And then do some one-armed press-ups. Oh yeah. Feeling the burn.

what you need
2 apples
½ a banana
4 ready-to-eat stoned prunes (man)
A spoonful of honey
A pinch of grated nutmeg
A dollop of natural yoghurt

what to do
Cut the apples into wedges, put them through the juicer and pour the juice into the blender. Add the banana, the prunes and the honey to the blender. Grate a generous sprinkling of nutmeg (or use the already-grated stuff if you can't be bothered) into the mixture along with a dollop of yoghurt and pulse twice. 2 servings.

As if you didn't know, prunes are very rich in fibre and help to keep bowel movements regular.

off to the small room you go.

the innocent foundation

We're giving 10% of the profits from this book (and all of the drinks we sell) to the innocent foundation (www.innocentfoundation.org). Here's a bit more about the NGOs and projects that the foundation supports:

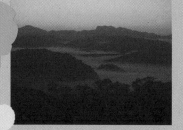

Iracambi

Iracambi's aim is to protect Brazil's Atlantic rainforest by making its conservation more attractive than its destruction to the local community.

Send a Cow

...isn't just about sending cows. It's more about enabling rural African communities to run small farms sustainably, with training in the arts of well construction, veg gardening and livestock husbandry.

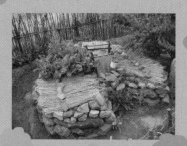

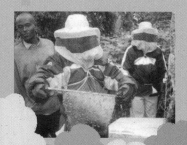

KIDA

This is a project that we completed in 2005, supporting eight villages to becoming self sufficient in bee-keeping. They now make lots of honey.

Find Your Feet

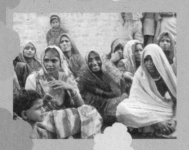

Our money is funding a project working with a community of 900 women in the Raibareli district of India, which hopes to improve access to water and promote sustainable farm practices.

CHICKS

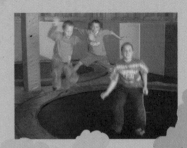

Country Holidays for Inner City Kids helps children who wouldn't otherwise get the chance to go on holiday in the countryside.

Groundwork West London

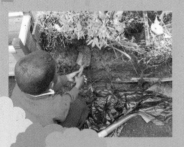

Groundwork provides environmental regeneration in deprived areas. We're supporting a project down the road at Berrymede Infant School, where Groundwork and the pupils are replanting the school grounds.

PLAN

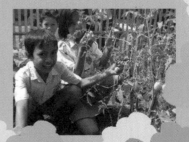

This charity educates schoolchildren in poor rural areas of Indonesia about the merits of organic farming.

orange and peach soya shake

It's a sad fact that these days, quite a lot of people seem to be lactose intolerant. The good news comes in the form of this drink, made using soya milk instead of yoghurt. And it tastes real nice to boot. NB As you may have read earlier, try to find soya milk that's made from the bean (not from isolates), and look out for any additives that shouldn't be there.

what you need
1 ½ oranges
150ml soya milk
3 peaches

what to do
Squeeze the juice from the oranges and pour into the blender. Remove the stones from the peaches, chop the flesh into chunks and add to the blender. Add the soya milk and whizz together until blended. 2 servings.

Liven this drink up with a sprinkling of oats or perhaps by passing 240volts through it.

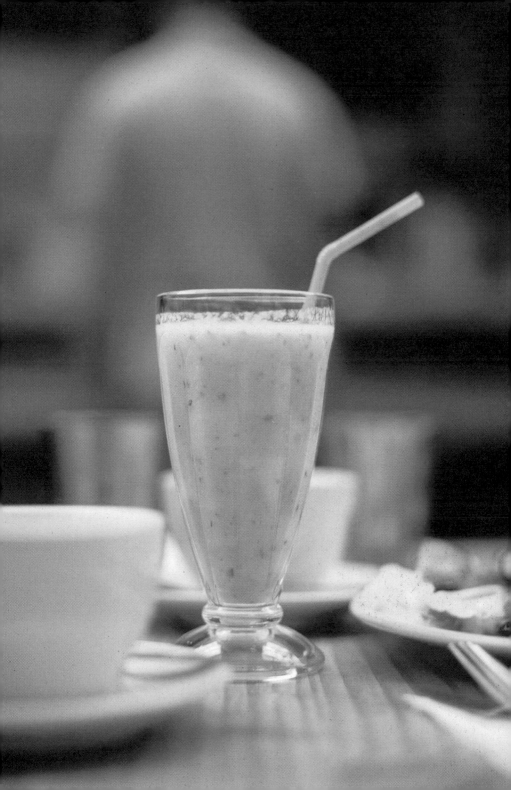

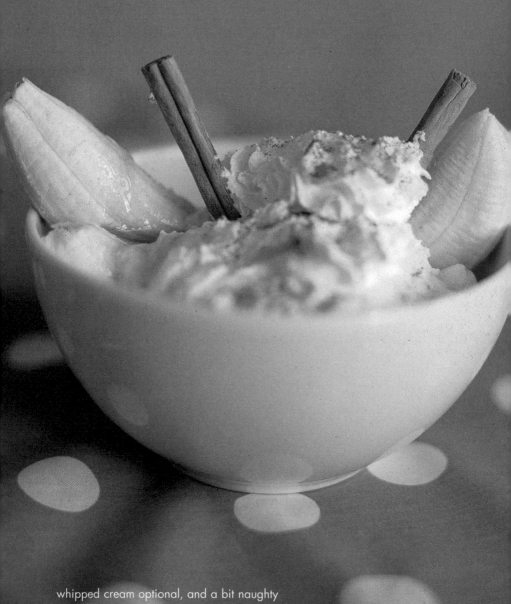

whipped cream optional, and a bit naughty

banana and cinnamon soya shake

Banana and cinnamon has been a favourite recipe at Fruit Towers since the dinosaurs walked the Earth, i.e. for quite a long time. We usually make it with yoghurt and a splash of apple juice, but this time we've gone for straight soya, making it a tad lighter. Still tastes special.

what you need
1 large banana
250ml of soya milk
2 tablespoons of honey
A touch of cinnamon

what to do
Peel and chop the banana and put it into the blender along with the soya milk and honey. Whizz until smooth. Serve with a sprinkling of cinnamon. 2 servings.

If you don't like soya milk, try using rice milk instead, or even good old-fashioned cow's milk.

veggies

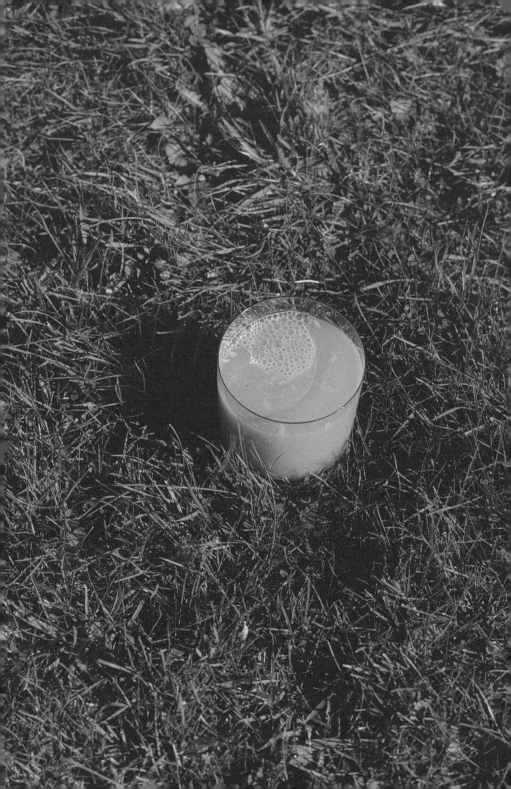

carrot, apple and ginger

This recipe was in our last book, but we're not ashamed to air it again. Put simply, it's the best veggie blend in all the world, and if anyone disagrees, we can sort it out in the car park at half seven.

what you need
3 carrots
2 apples
A chunk of fresh ginger

what to do
Scrub the carrots, then top and tail them. Cut the apples into wedges and put them and the carrots through the juicer. Mix the apple and carrot juice in a jug. Peel and finely grate a chunk (1–2cm) of ginger into the jug. Stir and serve. 1 serving.

Carrots are amazing. They're the richest vegetable source of vitamin A. What's more, drinking carrot juice allows you to absorb the good bits (carotenoids) more easily than if you ate the carrots.

broccoli, pear and kiwi

The mere mention of the word broccoli may scare some of you off. But please don't hide in the wardrobe. Broccoli is your friend. It contains as much calcium as milk, pound for pound, and lots of fibre and vitamin C as well. It's a nutrient powerhouse. But if you're still feeling nervous, please note – you can't really taste it in this recipe.

what you need
2 apples
1 pear
2 broccoli florets
2 kiwis (the fruit, that is. The birds don't taste so good.)

what to do
Cut the apples and pear into wedges, put them through the juicer and then pour the juice into the blender. Juice the broccoli florets and add this juice to the blender as well. Cut the kiwis in half and scoop the flesh into the blender. Give everything a quick whizz. Enjoy. 2 servings.

One kiwi fruit contains as much vitamin C as two oranges.

Cor, well I never.

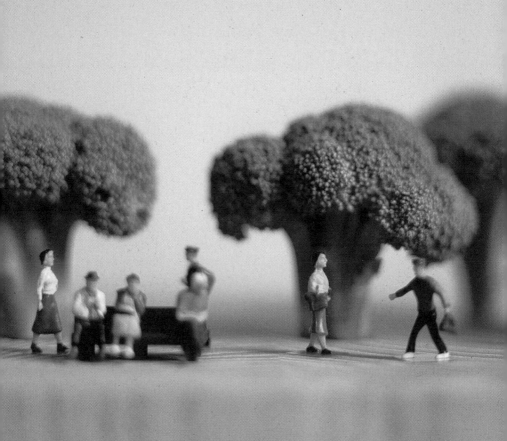

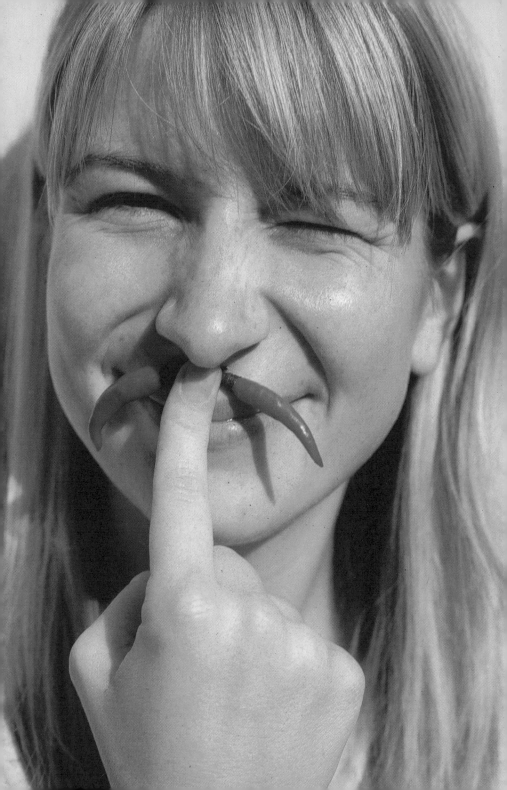

baby beetroot and chilli

Not your everyday juice. But that shouldn't stop you from making it. One blast of this chap and you'll be dancing the hornpipe, or something. What we're trying to say is that it tastes great, is quite hot (chilli hot) and outrageously good for you. If you're feeling lucky, leave the seeds in when you juice the chilli.

what you need
4 raw baby beets
2 apples
1 nice, spicy red chilli

what to do
Wash the baby beets, cut into wedges and put them through the juicer. Cut the apple into wedges and put them through the juicer. Deseed the chilli and put it through the juicer. (We used one of those large red chillies – the small ones are a bit more pokey, so please take care.) Mix all of the juices together in a big jug, stir and serve. 2 servings.

To get rid of the chilli taste from your juices, put a lemon (without shiny peel) through it. It'll naturally clean things up.

and for our next trick...

...we will show you some other ways to get fruit and veg into your diet without really noticing. Of course, you could just chop up some healthy stuff and hide it in your club sandwich, but there are many other ways to get the job done:

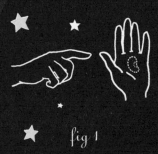

Chuck some beans in your curry, put some peas in with your pasta and make some fancy guacamole by smushing up some avocados, lime juice and chillies.

fig 1

A bowl of cereal is naked without some blueberries or bananas on top.

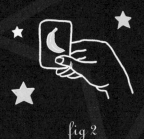

fig 2

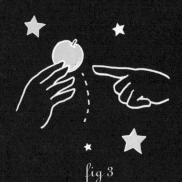

fig 3

Don't eat crisps. Just leave them. Bet yourself you can live for a week without them, and win the bet by eating an apple every time a pack of Walkers comes into your field of vision.

Buy some dried fruit and stick it on your desk. It won't go off, unlike that green tangerine you've been cultivating. You know, the one that lives in the mug with the coffee dregs.

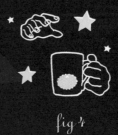

fig 4

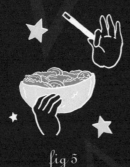

fig 5

If you're having a kebab, get the nice kebab man to stuff it full of salad and toms. Abra Kebabra. There you go.

PS don't get the doner — we've seen that thing on TV where they show them 'making' the meat. Risky.

Get your boss to buy a blender for the kitchen at work. Kettles are so last year.

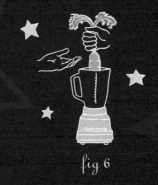

fig 6

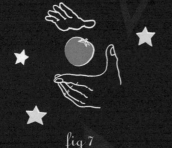

fig 7

Erm, chop up some tomatoes and salad and stick them in your club sandwich.

If you're doing all of this (and drinking the odd smoothie) you'll be getting your five a day without even noticing. And remember, fresh is obviously best, but please don't be scared to eat frozen, dried or tinned stuff. It all counts.

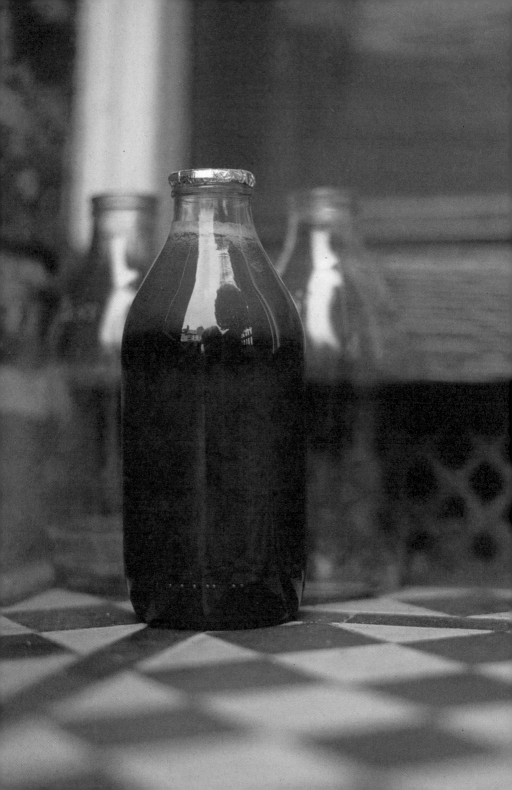

carrot, beetroot and celery

Ever wondered why your milkman's so happy in the morning? Well, it might have something to do with the fact that he drank one of these before he came out to do his rounds, making him feel as perky as a badger. Could also have something to do with the fact that his working day finishes at 9.30am.

what you need
2 carrots
1 raw beetroot (or 2 baby ones)
1 stick of celery
1 apple

what to do
Cut everything into bits and put them through the juicer, apples last. Stir and serve. 1 serving.

apple, spinach and nutmeg

Nutmeg – ancient spice, mild hallucinogen (if you eat about three tons of it) and saviour of rubbish rice puddings. We are honoured by your presence.

what you need
2 apples
1 large handful of spinach leaves
A generous sprinkling of grated nutmeg

what to do
Cut the apples into wedges and put them through the juicer. Wash and destalk the spinach leaves and put them through the juicer. Grate a generous sprinkling of nutmeg into the juice and stir. 1 serving.

Use baby spinach if possible, as you don't really have to destalk it.

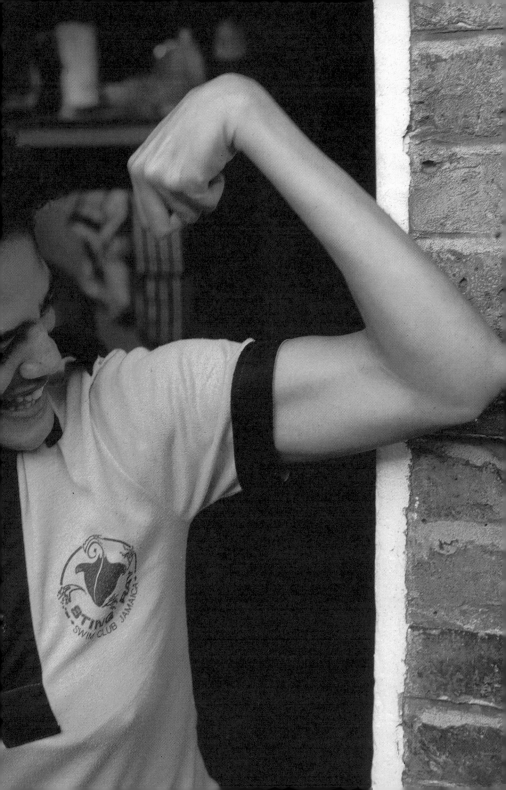

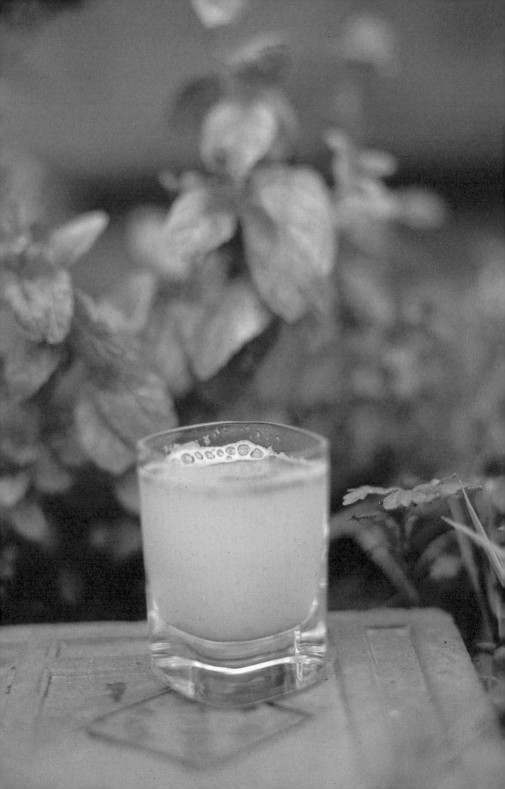

celery, apple and mint

Mint's pretty easy to grow. Just buy some at the garden centre and transplant it into your backyard when you get the chance. Then you'll have fresh mint for this recipe any time you need it. How convenient.

what you need
2 crunchy apples
1 stick of celery
Some fresh mint

what to do
Cut the apples into wedges, put them through the juicer and pour juice into the blender. Juice the celery stick and add the juice to the blender, along with a sprig of fresh mint. Blend and serve. 1 serving.

Don't use Murray mints instead of fresh mint.
You'll muck up your blender.

juices

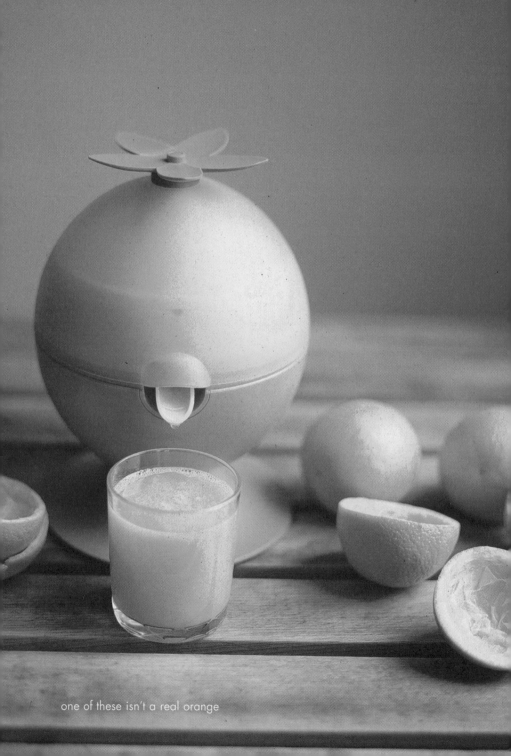

one of these isn't a real orange

orange, mango and lime

We kind of did this one the wrong way round. We came up with the recipe, tested it out in the shops for a couple of years and then finally decided that it was good enough for our recipe book. Anyway, we hope you enjoy it.

what you need
¼ of a mango
3 oranges
A wedge of lime

what to do
Peel the mango, remove the stone and chop the flesh into pieces. Squeeze the oranges, add the OJ to the blender with the mango pieces and squeeze in some lime juice. Blend, serve, drink. 1 generous serving.

If you throw a lime at your brother, it could hurt him.

cucumber, orange and mint

Healthy fast food is the holy grail as far as we're concerned. So we were chuffed when we found a real healthy fast food place right here in London, called Leon. We thought it was only right and proper to give them a ring and see if they fancied chipping in a recipe. Luckily they did. So here's one that Allegra (chief Leon recipe person) sent over. It tastes mighty good, as you might expect.

what you need
1 apple
1 cucumber
3 oranges
A small bunch of fresh mint

what to do
Cut the apple into wedges and the cucumber into chunks and put them both through the juicer. Squeeze the oranges. Put all of the juice into the blender with the mint leaves and give it a thorough whizz. 2 servings.

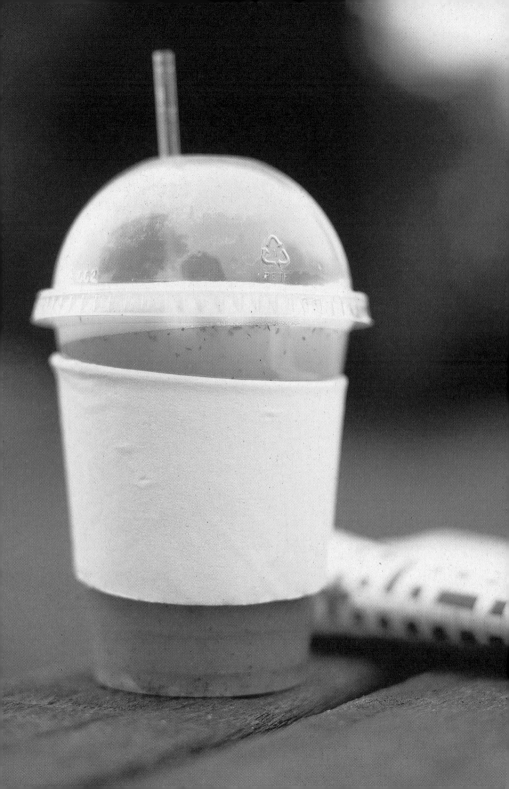

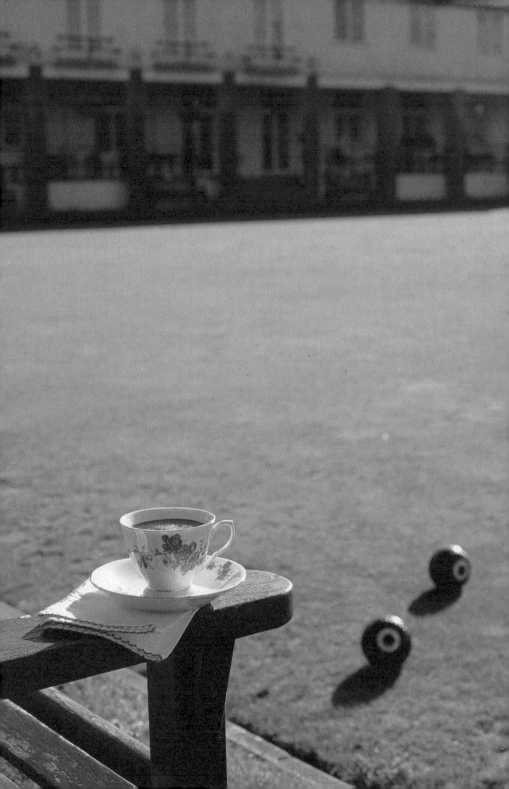

apple, blackcurrant and elderflower

We say yes to proper deckchairs. Manicured lawns. Net curtains. Well-trimmed moustaches. These are the things that make us feel proud to be British. Along with this very British drink.

what you need
2 apples
20 blackcurrants
3 teaspoons of elderflower cordial

what to do
Cut the apples into wedges and put them through the juicer. Put the apple juice, blackcurrants and elderflower cordial into the blender and whizz until smooth. Sing 'Rule Britannia'. Drink. 1 serving.

Elderflowers have magic powers. Pop a sprig in your hat to ward off midges and deter surprise caterpillar attacks by putting bruised elder leaves around your little budding plants.

X marks the spot

It's about this time in our recipe books that we like to stop and think about camping. We love camping.

Our camping trips work like this. We leave work at noon on Friday. This gives us time to get as far as possible from town, up to our favourite spot in a deserted dale. In no time at all we've pitched our tents, built a fire and are sitting around talking nonsense. Cooking outdoors, sleeping under the stars, going for big long walks and eating rabbit pie for lunch. Life doesn't get much better. Well, maybe a loo would help. Those ferns sure do tickle.

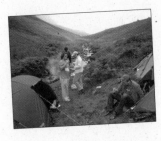

Anyway, if you fancy finding out where our secret spot is, you can email us. If we reckon you'll take care of it and keep it a secret, we'll let you know where it is.

Send enquiries to:
thespecialplace@innocentdrinks.co.uk

…and don't forget your head-torch.

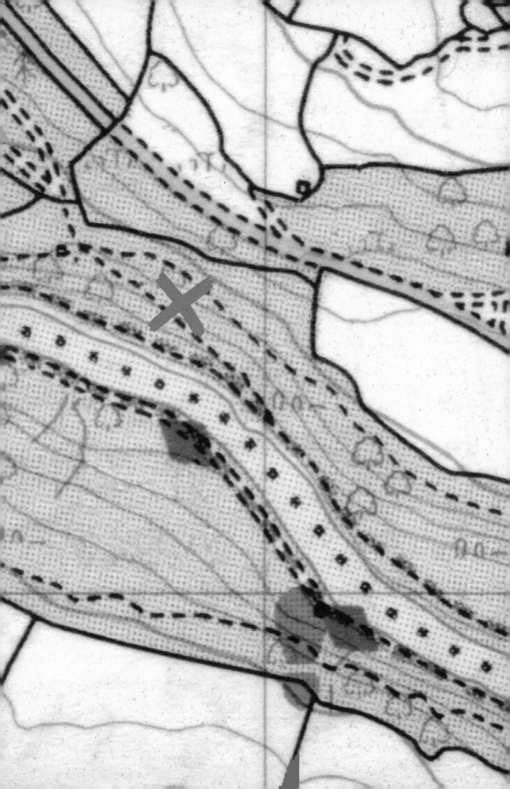

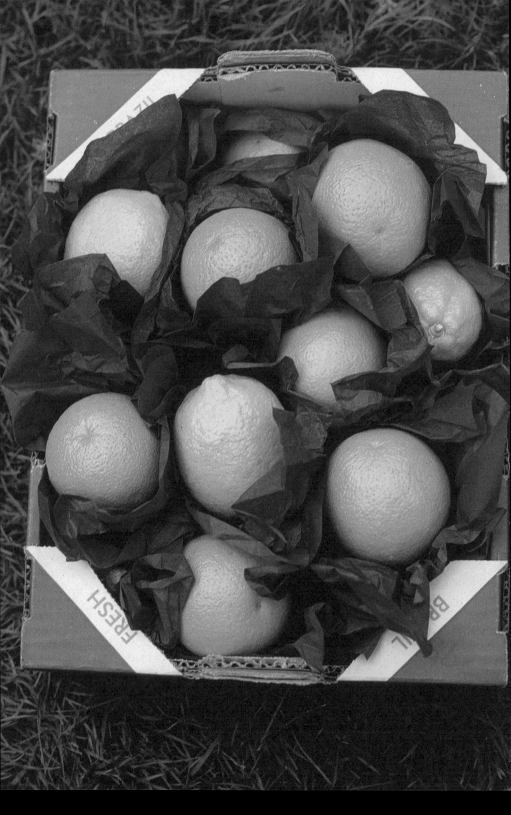

st clements

Oranges and lemons
Say the bells of St Clements
Chuck in some grapefruit
Say the bells of St, erm, Grapefruit

what you need
2 oranges
1½ pink grapefruits
½ a lemon

what to do
Squeeze the juice from the oranges and grapefruits into a jug. Add a squeeze of lemon and give everything a good stir. Relax, drink, enjoy and add ice if you're feeling a little hot. 2 servings.

If you're looking for vitamin C, this is the mothership. Vit C helps keeps your skin and bones healthy, so drink it all down.

the cardigan bay kickstart

The good people at howies sent us this recipe. howies are based in Cardigan Bay and they make great clothes and other useful stuff. They also have an ethos that we admire – you should check them out at howies.co.uk. Anyway, their recipe is pretty amazing – a sort of power juice with ginger and seaweed. It'll get you cranking in the morning, that's for sure.

what you need
1 teaspoon of arame seaweed
3 apples
1 lemon
A chunk of fresh ginger

what to do
Pre-soak the seaweed according to the pack instructions. Cut the apples into wedges, put them through the juicer and pour the juice into the blender. Squeeze the lemon juice into the blender. Peel and finely grate a nice chunk (1–2cm) of ginger and chuck it into the blender along with the seaweed. Drink and feel strangely powerful. 1 serving.

You can get arame seaweed at most decent health food stores. Don't use seaweed that you found down at the beach.

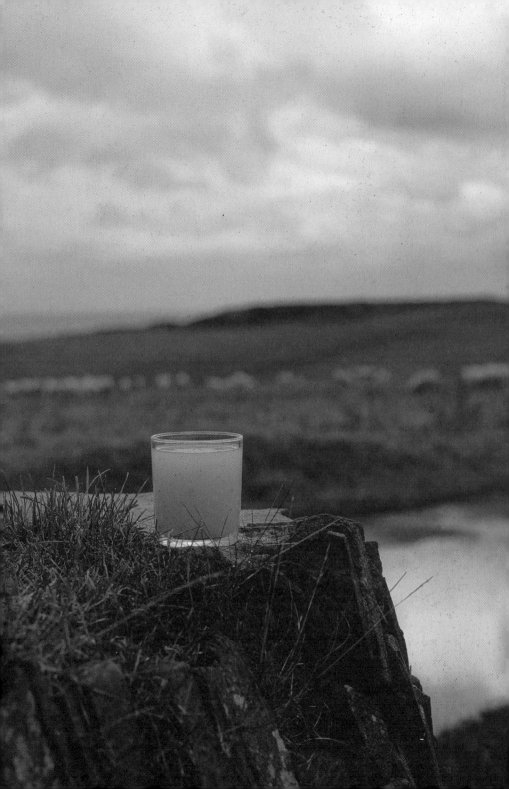

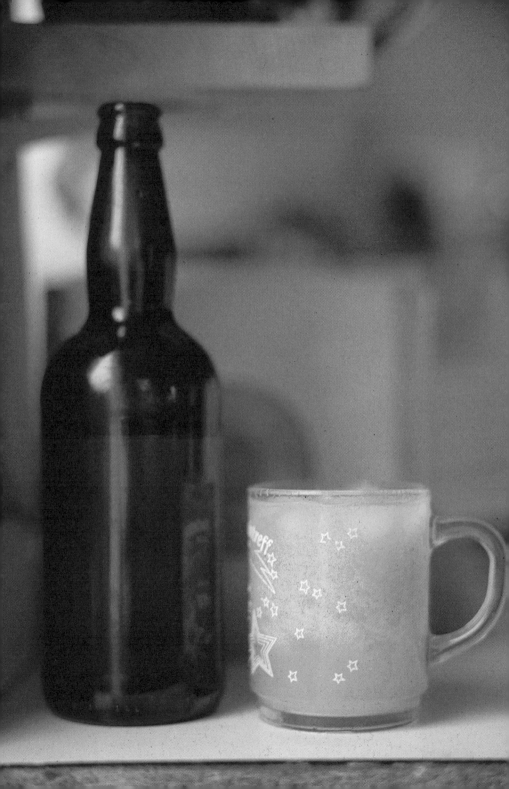

ginger beer and mango

If we'd put a superfluous comma in this recipe title, it would have read ginger, beer and mango. Then we would have had a situation where the recipe would have included some ginger, a can of Hofmeister and a bit of mango. It is on such tiny details that the world can change – a butterfly flaps its wings in Japan and we end up with lager in our juice. Just shows that it's worth learning your grammar.

what you need
½ a mango
A handful of ice cubes
1 can/bottle of strong ginger beer (ice cold)

what to do
Peel and chop the mango into little chunks. Put them in the blender and whizz until the mango is smooth. Pour the ginger beer into a tall ice-filled glass and stir in the mango pulp with your favourite spoon. 1 generous serving.

Ginger beer contains a very small amount of alcohol. Enough to get a beetle drunk, probably.

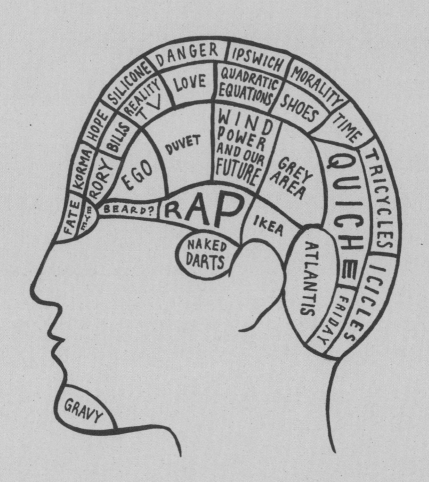

Mental Interlude

OK, so this bit doesn't have much to do with making nice drinks. But we think it all comes from the same place – a desire to do ourselves a bit of good, to ensure that our lives are a little bit better and longer.

And so it follows that the mental side of things is just as important as the physical, nutritional stuff you do to yourself. So we'd like to take a moment to pass on some thoughts about how you can give your brain a break:

Have a nap
We could learn a lot from our Spanish brothers and sisters – short naps really do work. Even 30 minutes is long enough to recharge the batteries.

Never eat lunch at your desk
Give yourself a full hour at lunchtime. Go to the park, sit on a bench and watch the squirrels.

Collect pine cones
It'll mean you get down to the woods more often, and it seems to make the squirrels happy.

Unplug your TV and turn off your phone
Just do it, even if it's only for one evening a week. Read, cook, play carpet golf, anything. Just lose the gadgets.

Go camping
See page 118.

lemon, manuka honey and ginger

Here's a fine drink for fighting a cold – a hot toddy, innocent style. We use Manuka honey because of its anti-bacterial properties, but regular honey will do. If you really want to up the ante, you can add a sprig of rosemary to further enhance its healthy powers.

what you need

1 unwaxed lemon
An inch of fresh ginger
6 teaspoons of Manuka honey
Boiling water from the kettle (approx 300ml)
A sprig of rosemary (totally optional)

what to do

Squeeze half the lemon and pour the juice into a mug. Slice the other half of the lemon. Finely slice the ginger. Add the lemon slices, honey and the ginger to the mug. (If you're adding rosemary, give it a quick bash with a rolling pin to release the oils and drop it in the mug now.) Pour on the boiling water. Leave to infuse and cool for 5 minutes. 2 servings.

For that true hot toddy effect, add a shot of brandy when no one's looking.

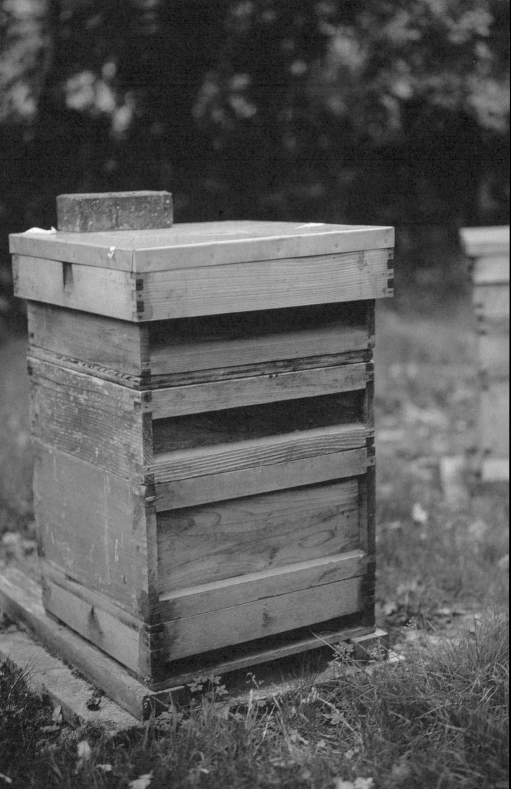

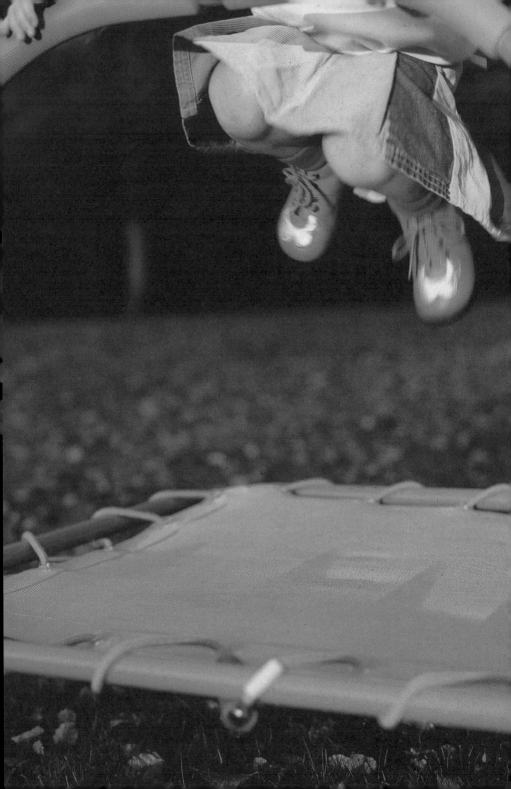

cranberry and orange

This is a really simple juice, but it can't be beaten for its sharp yet sweet taste, nor for the amount of good it'll do you. We urge everybody to get more cranberries into their lives, not least because they keep our waterworks in good running order. We feel that this is quite important.

what you need
2 apples
2 oranges
50g of cranberries

what to do
Cut the apple into wedges and put them through the juicer. Freshly squeeze two oranges. Add the orange juice, apple juice and cranberries to the blender and whizz until mixed. 2 servings.

Cranberry growers bounce their cranberries to see if they are good enough to sell. Good ones bounce, bad ones don't.

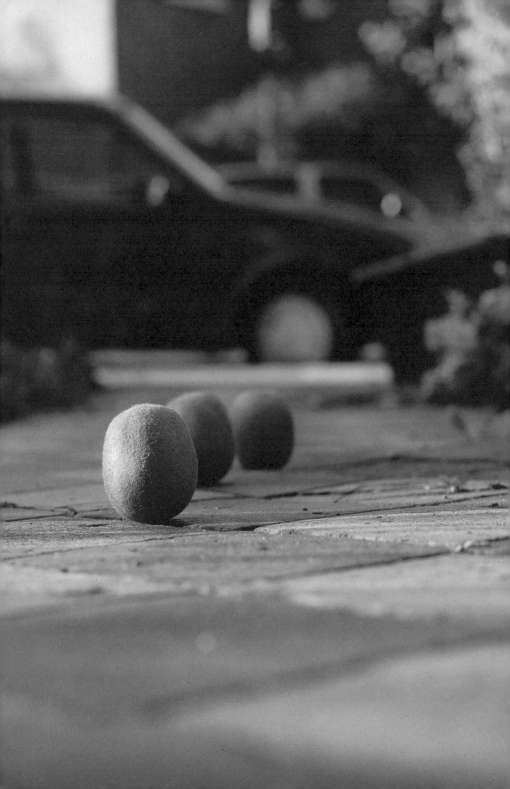

kiwi and lime

We've been drinking this at Fruit Towers for years. But we've struggled to get it into the shops. You see, kiwi misbehaves. It doesn't seem to like being in bottles. We're still working on it, but for now you're going to have to make it yourselves.

what you need
1½ apples
A small bunch of green grapes
3 kiwis
The juice and zest of half a lime

what to do
Cut the apples into wedges and put them through the juicer. Put the grapes through the juicer too. Peel the kiwi fruits. Add the apple juice, grape juice, a squeeze of lime juice and the lime zest to the blender. Whizz thoroughly before adding the kiwis, then pulse briefly until smooth. 2 servings.

Don't blend the kiwis too much or the seeds get broken and taste peppery. Grape skin can also taste bitter, so see if you can get someone to peel them for you.

posh stuff

mango and pistachio

We remember a time when pistachios didn't exist. In fact, we're sure that the only nut we ever used to see was the peanut, and that was usually in the pub. So we reckon that somewhere out there is the person who invented pistachios, probably around 1986. If you know who it is, please let us know – call the banana phone on 020 8600 3939.

what you need
1 mango
2 apples
3 tablespoons of bio-yoghurt
1 teaspoon of honey
30g of unsalted pistachio nuts

what to do
Peel the mango and slice it into the blender. Cut the apples into wedges, put them through the juicer and pour the juice into the blender. Whizz until smooth. Add the yoghurt and honey to the blender. Pulse 4 times. Coarsely crush up some pistachios in a pestle and mortar (or mini food processor) and sprinkle them on the top. 2 servings.

If you're lazy like us, buy shelled pistachios. Much easier on the nails. And make sure they're unsalted.

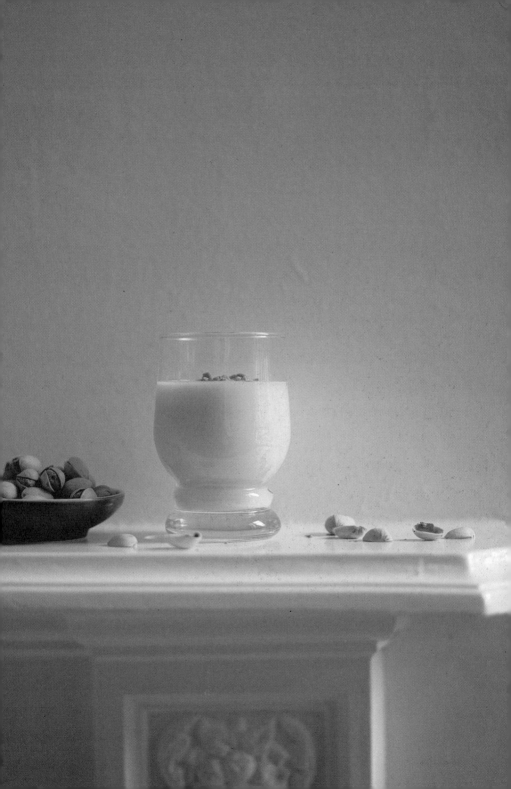

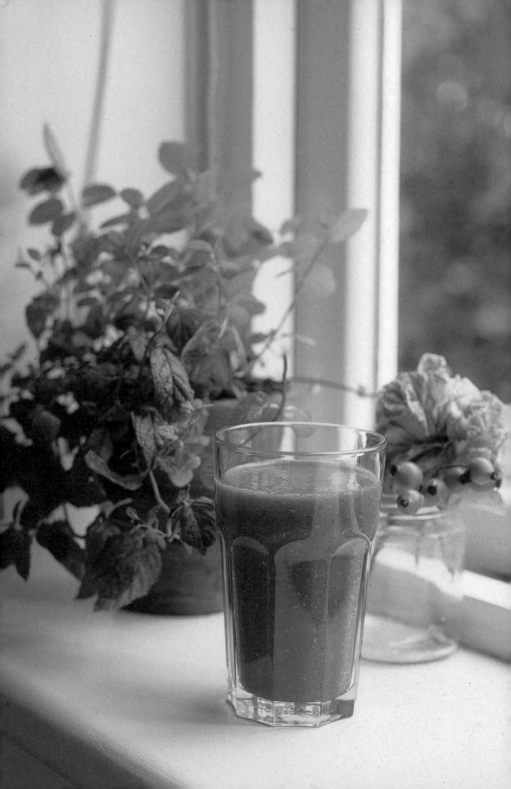

raspberry and roses

This one's for lovers. Make it for your sweetheart first thing in the morning and their day will be rose-scented. Or save it for Valentine's Day breakfast and decorate with rose petals. You soppy thing.

what you need
2 apples
1 orange
1 punnet of raspberries
½ a banana
1 dessertspoon of rose water (or one teaspoon of rose syrup if you can get it)

what to do
Cut the apples into wedges, put them through the juicer and pour the juice into the blender. Squeeze the juice from the orange. Add the orange juice to the blender, along with the raspberries, banana and rose water/syrup. Whizz. Drink. Fall in love. 2 servings.

We got our le Jardin d'Elen rose Syrup from La fromagerie, a posh London cheese shop. But you can get rose water in supermarkets, in the aisle with the glacé cherries and baking ingredients.

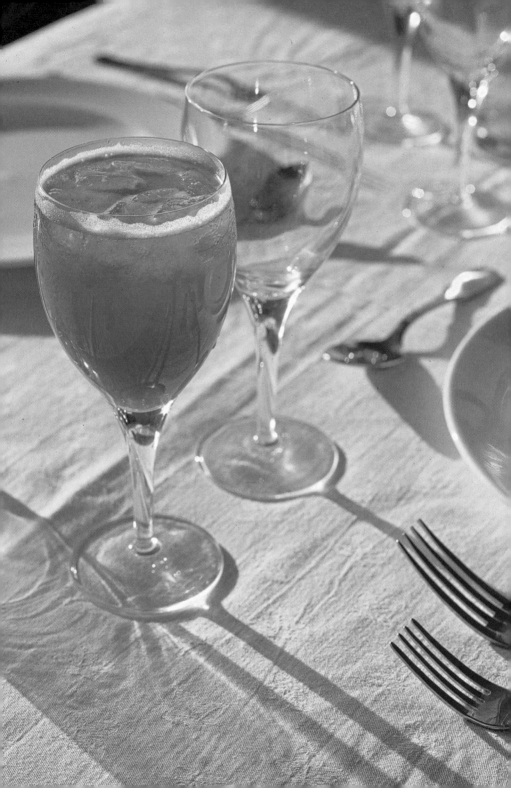

watermelon and hibiscus iced tea

If this drink was a person, it would live in Kensington, buy groceries at Fortnum and Mason and could well own a beagle. In short, it's a bit posh, and none the worse for it.

what you need
⅛ of a watermelon
200ml of cold hibiscus tea (made with 3 teaspoons of dried hibiscus flowers)
100ml of soda water
A wedge of lime
1 teaspoon of sugar
6 ice cubes

what to do
Remove and discard the rind and seeds from the watermelon. Chop the flesh into chunks, place in the blender and whizz. Pour the cold tea into a tall glass and add the watermelon puree, soda water, lime juice and sugar. Stir gently. Add the ice cubes, give a final stir and serve. 3 servings.

Get dried hibiscus flowers from a health food store. And don't use hibiscus flowers from your garden; your stomach won't like them.

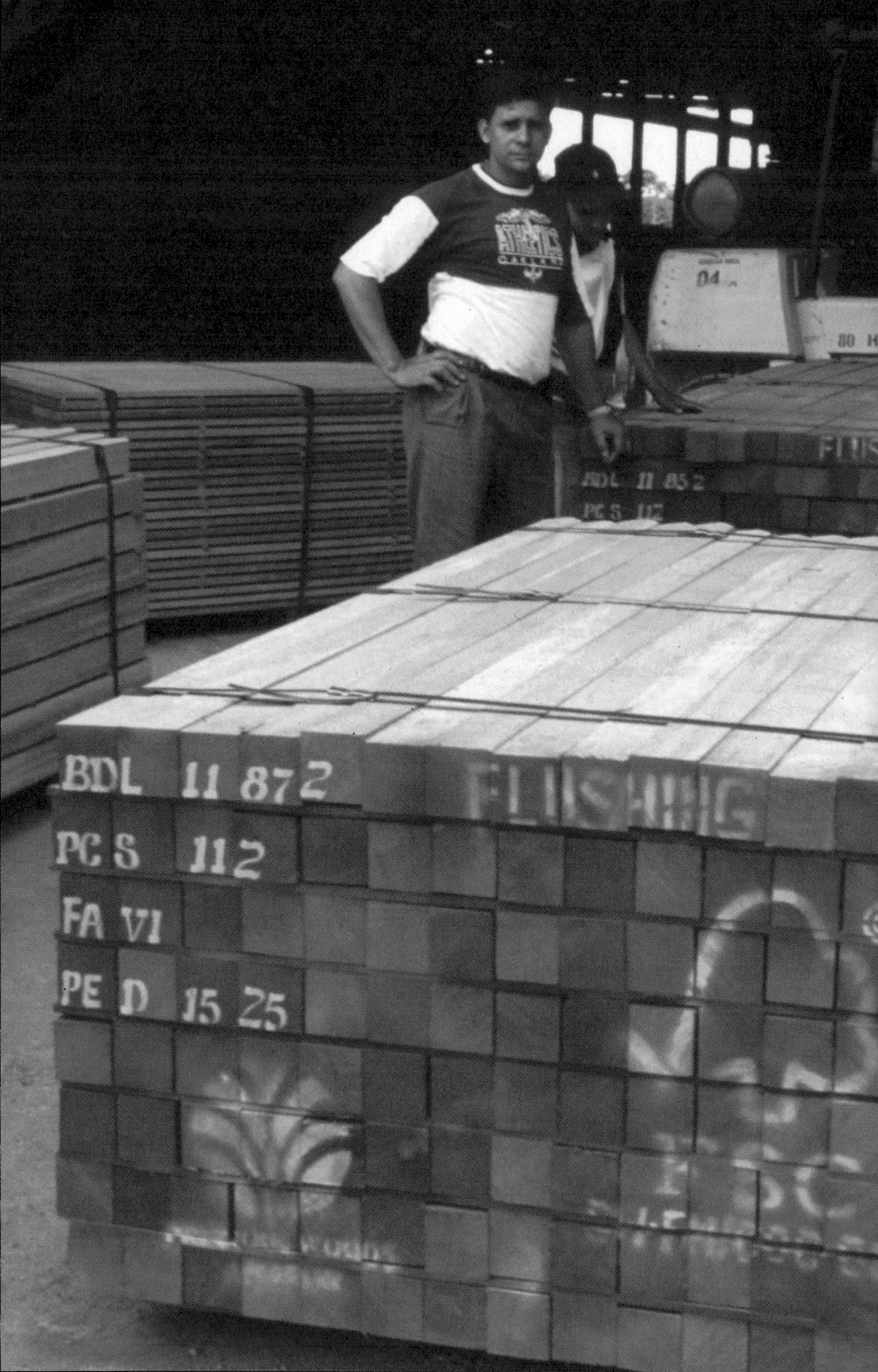
BDL 11 87 2
PC S 112
FA VI
PE D 15 25
FLUSHING

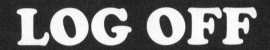

LOG OFF

Over the past 30 years 15% of the Brazilian Amazon rainforest has been completely destroyed (an area the size of France). This is not a good thing. Deforestation decreases rainfall in the area and contributes to global warming, which in turn dries out the rainforest and causes it to die back. Still not a good thing.

Now, we're all vaguely aware of this. But in our modern age of Wi-Fi kettles and robot dogs, we seem to have become distracted, and have forgotten that saving the rainforest is a pretty good idea and is quite straightforward. We can all do a bit to help:

1 Only buy wood and wood products that have been certified by the Forest Stewardship Council (FSC). Look for their logo or ask the store manager.

2 Animal feed for poultry, pigs and cows (for dairy products as well as beef) is usually soya based. Lots of cheap soya is grown on recently cleared rainforest land. So make sure that the meat you buy is organic, as organic feed doesn't contain 'bad' soya. In other words, cut back on cheap burgers.

3 If you use products containing soya, find out where the soya comes from. Phone the number on the pack/carton to ask and avoid any soya that comes from the Amazon region of Brazil.

Find out more at www.greenpeace.org.uk/forests

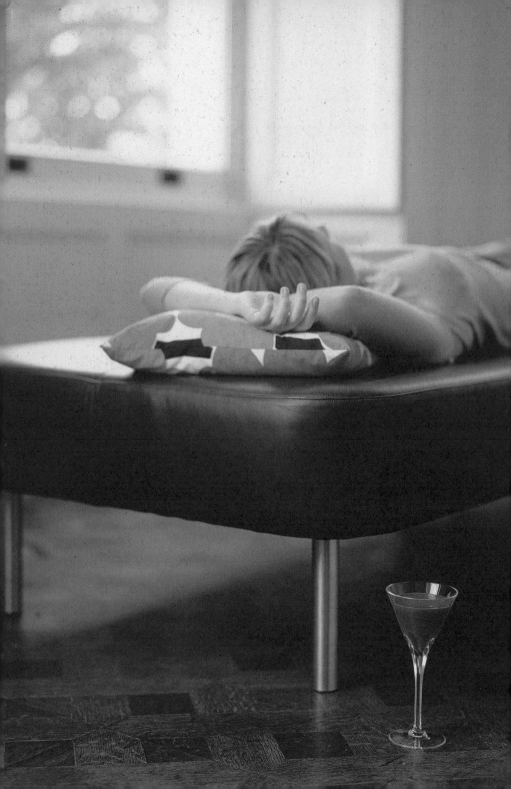

dark chocolate and cherry

For those moments in life when only the best will do. Lie on the sofa, switch on the telly and watch a French film with subtitles or perhaps a fancy programme about Renaissance art. You know, something a bit classy. Obviously, there should be someone else in the kitchen making you one of these.

what you need
2 apples
10 cherries
½ a banana
50g of dark chocolate

what to do
Cut the apples into wedges, put them through the juicer and pour the juice into the blender. Chop up the cherries, discarding the stones. Slice the banana and add it and the cherries to the blender. Whizz everything together. Melt the chocolate in a bowl set over a pan of simmering water. Add the melted chocolate to the blended ingredients and give it all a final whizz. 2 servings.

Use morello cherries to make this taste even better. And don't feel guilty - dark chocolate contains antioxidants that help to lower blood pressure.

strawberry, meringue and crème fraîche

Paul, an innocent drinker, sent us in this recipe. He says 'I have tried it out on my friends and they think it's ace.' There can be no higher recommendation.

what you need
10 strawberries
150ml of semi-skimmed milk
3 tablespoons of crème fraîche
½ a small meringue
Mint sprigs to serve

what to do
Pop the strawberries into the blender with the milk and crème fraîche and blend. Put the blended mixture into a glass, crumble in the meringue and stir gently. 2 servings.

Decorate with half a strawberry and a sprig of mint if you're trying to impress someone.

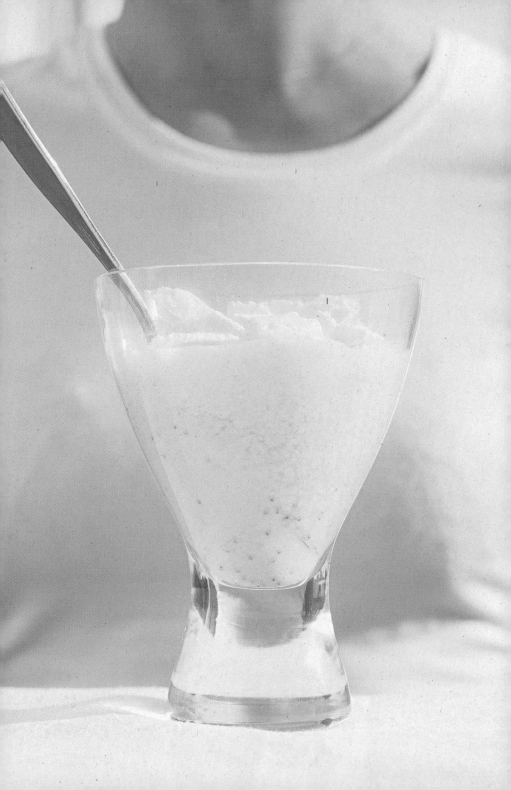

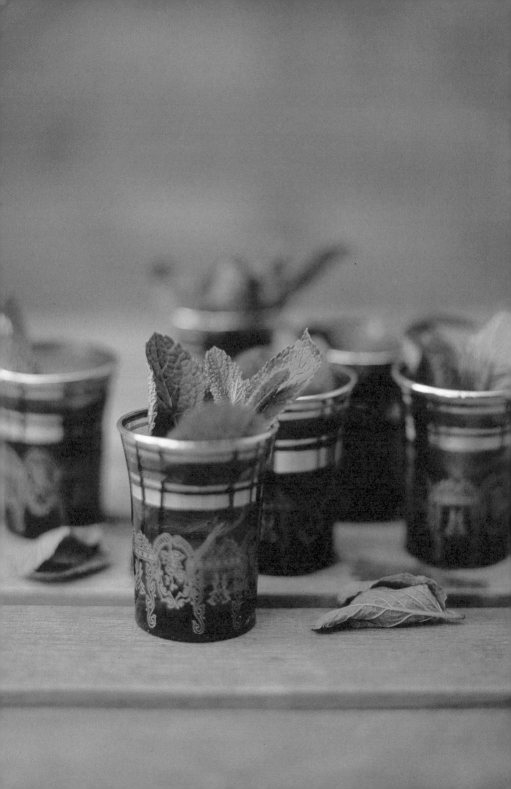

moroccan mint tea

Our Lucy went off to Morocco for a bit of fun in the sun and came back with this recipe. She brought back a teapot and those little cups too.

what you need
Green tea
Boiling water
A large handful of fresh mint
Sugar to taste
A teapot

what to do
Brew the green tea as per pack instructions (enough for two cups) in your teapot. Add the mint to the teapot at the end of the brewing (don't add it before or it'll taste nasty). Add a touch of sugar to taste. Pour from a great height, like they do in Morocco. 2 servings.

You could use white tea instead of green tea for a stronger antioxidant effect. And if you're using a proper Moroccan teapot, be careful of the hot handle.

the innocent wee-ometer™

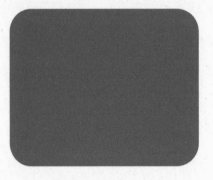

A night out with Keith Richards.

Office party.

No one can see the smell of asparagus.

Half a shandy.

Smoothies and juices are great, but we all know you're supposed to drink a bit of water too. An easy way to check that you're getting enough water is to use our patented innocent wee-ometer™. Just compare your wee to what's on the chart – the darker your wee, the more water you need to drink. A nice pale yellow (Wee Nirvana®) is what you should be aiming for.

"Blow into the bag please Sir."

Beetroot surprise.

Wee Nirvana®.

I can pee clearly now.

mango and basil

Bored one day in Cardiff, Jo and Andrew (two innocent drinkers) decided to come up with this recipe. Praise be for boredom.

what you need
2 apples
1 ripe mango
A wedge of lime
A large sprig of basil

what to do
Cut the apples into wedges, put them through the juicer and pour the juice into the blender. Peel and slice the mango into the blender. Add a squeeze of lime juice and a few fresh basil leaves. Whizz until well mixed. 2 servings.

Tips for keeping your shop-bought basil plant alive:
1. cut off sprigs that grow rapidly and shoot out
2. only water it when the leaves are wilting a bit
3. sing it some love songs - maybe Chris de Burgh

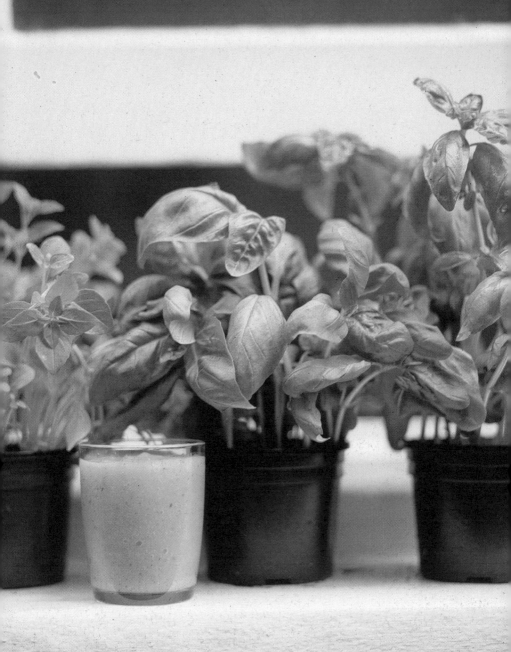

Basil, meet Basil

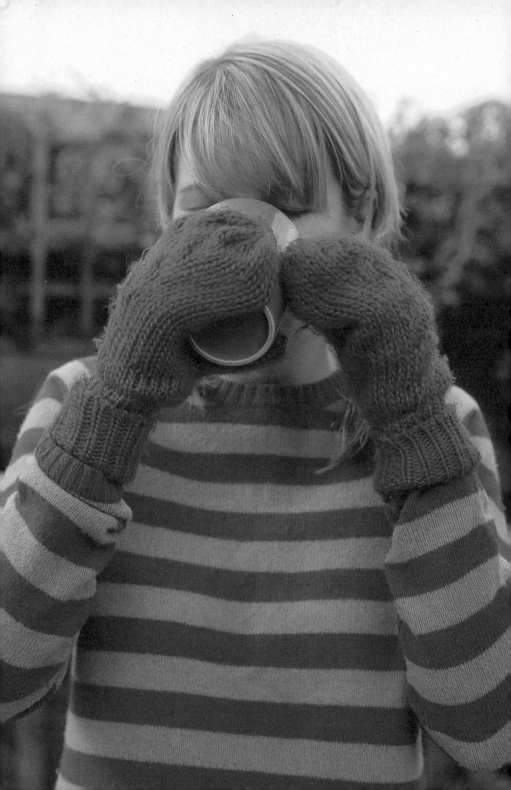

chocolate milk with pear and ginger

A nice person called Micah sent this recipe to us. Micah is in charge of developing new recipes at Green & Black's (the nice organic chocolate people), so we are kind of in awe, seeing as we eat so much of their stuff.

what you need
200ml of semi-skimmed milk
40g of Green & Black's 70% solid dark chocolate
1 ripe pear
½ a piece of crystallised stem ginger

what to do
In a small pan, gently heat the milk with the chocolate (broken into small pieces) until the chocolate has melted. Peel and core the pear and cut into quarters. Add the pear, chocolate milk and stem ginger to the blender and blend until smooth. Serve warm or chilled. 1 greedy serving.

kids' stuff

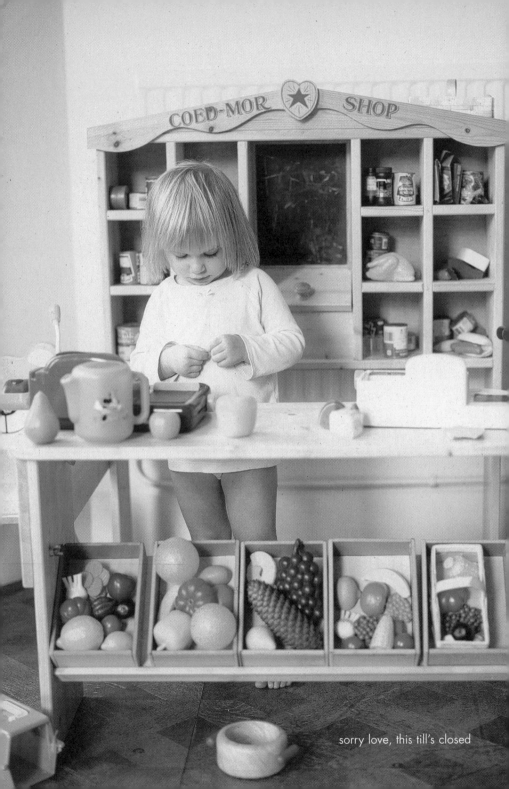

sorry love, this till's closed

kiwi and apple

Getting kids to eat fruit can sometimes feel like trying to get toothpaste back into the tube. But smoothies seem to work – when it's in a glass it suddenly becomes a bit more interesting. Like this recipe.

what you need
2½ apples
2 kiwis
½ an orange
½ a banana
A wedge of lemon

what to do
Cut the apples into wedges and put them through the juicer. Peel the kiwis and slice them into the blender. Squeeze the orange. Add the banana, the apple and orange juice and a squeeze of lemon juice to the blender. Whizz until smooth. 2 servings.

Always remember to put the lid on your blender, unless you're planning on redecorating soon.

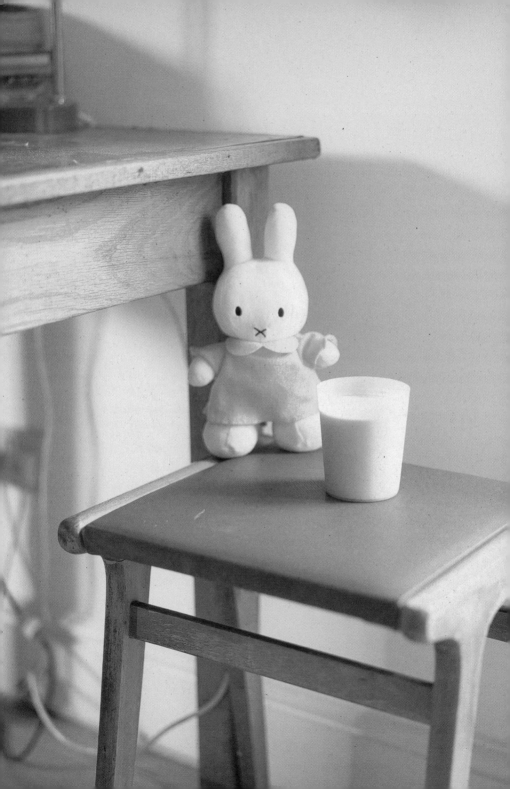

jamie oliver's mango and ginger smoothie

That nice Jamie Oliver has lent us one of his recipes for our book. Since he did his school dinners thing he has become a hero to thousands of parents, so we thought we should stick his recipe in our kids' section.

what you need
2 ripe mangoes
1 banana, peeled
A thumb-sized piece of ginger, peeled and finely grated
250ml of cold organic full-fat milk
250ml of cold organic apple juice
Optional: 1 vanilla pod (as a luxurious extra!)

what to do
Jamie's instructions are as follows:

'Before making this recipe, make sure your mangoes are ripe – you want those delicious ones that smell and taste like nectar. Peel the mangoes and then use your (clean) hands to squeeze and pull all the flesh away from the stone. Put the mango flesh and banana into your blender and whizz for 30 seconds. Add the grated ginger, milk and apple juice and, if you're using a vanilla pod, split it in half lengthways, scrape out the vanilla seeds and add those, too. (Don't throw away your empty vanilla pod – pop it in a bag of sugar to give it a delicious vanilla flavour.) Finally, whizz again until you have a lovely smoothie consistency. Serves 4.

'PS try putting a little bit of this smoothie into a bowl and serving it with a sprinkle of strawberries and some vanilla ice cream. A great summer's dessert.'

black apples

We were given this recipe by Lizzie Vann, the founder of Baby Organix. She says that this one is rich in iron – just the sort of thing to give your little 'uns to make sure they grow up big and strong.

what you need
2 apples
50 blackcurrants
2 apricots
1 teaspoon of black treacle

what to do
Cut the apples into wedges and put them through the juicer. Add the apple juice, the blackcurrants, stoned apricots and the treacle to the blender and whizz until smooth. 2 kids' servings.

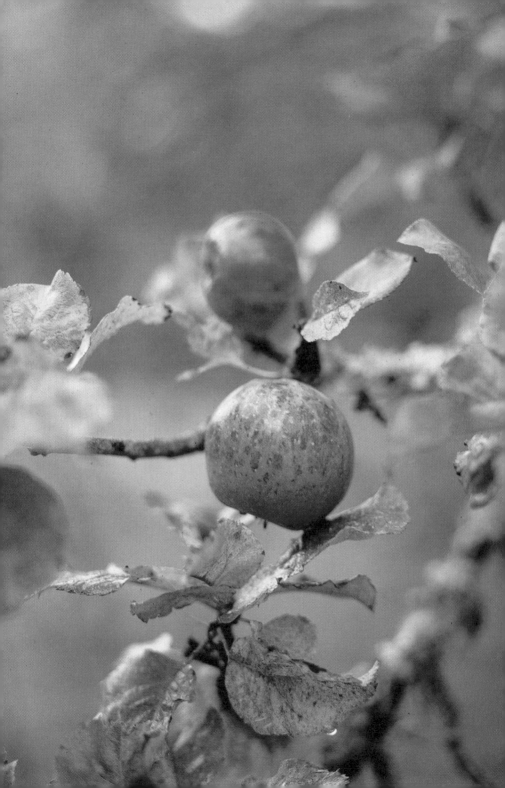

keep it tidy

The Earth is a finite resource. There's only one of them
and various bits of it seem to be being used up pretty
quickly. So we feel that we have a duty to leave things
a tiny bit better than we found them. You know, tidy our
rooms, wash the dishes and reduce all of the negative
impacts our business system has on the world.

Ultimately, we're aiming to be a 100% sustainable company,
and are trying to ensure that the way we do business
leaves a neutral or, better still, positive footprint on the
world around us. It'll take a bit of work, but hey, we
haven't got anything better to do.

To help reduce our impacts, we're focusing our long-term efforts in three main areas:

ingredients

We'll only work with fruit growers who treat their land and their employees well. So we say no to this lot – the use of harmful chemicals, the degradation of the local environment, bonded labour and anything else that damages the relationship between nature and communities. We also refuse to air-freight our ingredients, for pretty obvious reasons.

packaging

We're striving to use as little as possible of everything, and are moving to 0% virgin finite resources across the board, which means we're using more recycled materials. Every little step helps.

us

We've always used renewable energy at Fruit Towers, and are now starting to carbon offset any CO_2 emissions that come either directly or indirectly from what we do. We'll also be asking anyone who works with us to go green, as a condition of us entering into business with them. And we'll use 100% recycled paper when we make books.

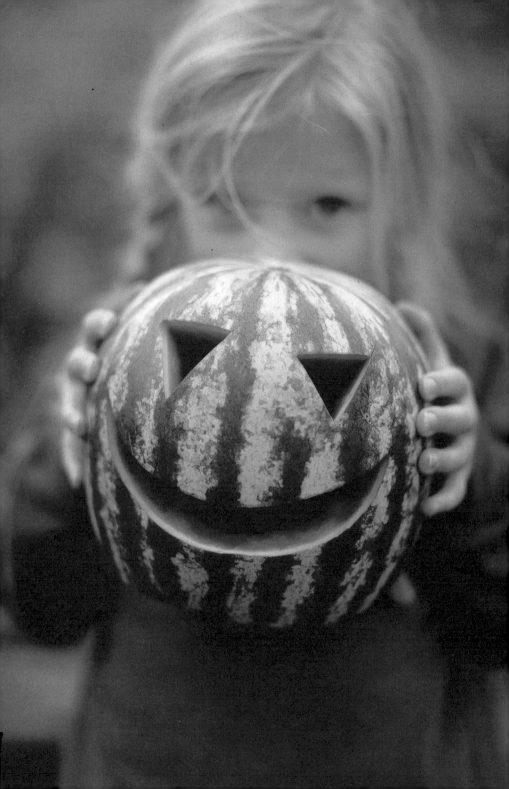

melon and berries

We are trying to invent a new fruit. It's called the melonberry. It's a bit like a melon but you can pop it into your mouth whole, like a berry. No peel, no seeds, just whole melonberry goodness. The problem is that it's quite difficult. The melon and the berry don't seem to want to mate. They're circling each other nervously and it looks like it might take a while. So we thought we'd make this recipe instead.

what you need
1 apple
½ a Galia melon
1 wedge of watermelon
½ a pink grapefruit
½ a banana
2 handfuls of frozen mixed berries

what to do
Cut the apple into wedges and put them through the juicer. Remove the seeds and skin from the melons, slice into wedges and put them through the juicer. Squeeze the grapefruit. Put the melon, apple and grapefruit juice into the blender with half a peeled banana and the berries and whizz until smooth. 2 servings.

You can use a whole Galia and no watermelon, but it does taste nicer if you use both.

raspberryade

There's bad fizzy pop and there's good fizzy pop. The bad stuff contains colouring, preservatives, sweeteners and other rubbish that kids don't need. The good stuff can be made at home from natural ingredients – see below.

what you need
1 punnet of raspberries
500ml of sparkling water
1 wedge of lemon
Sugar or honey to taste

what to do
Wash the raspberries and blitz them in a blender. Add the sparkling water and a squeeze of lemon juice and stir gently. Pass the mixture through a sieve to get rid of any seeds. Stir in a little sugar or honey to taste. 3 servings.

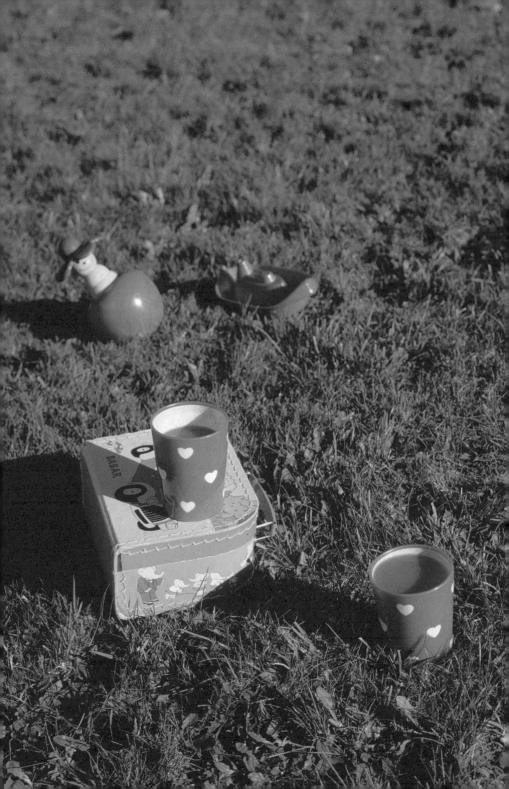

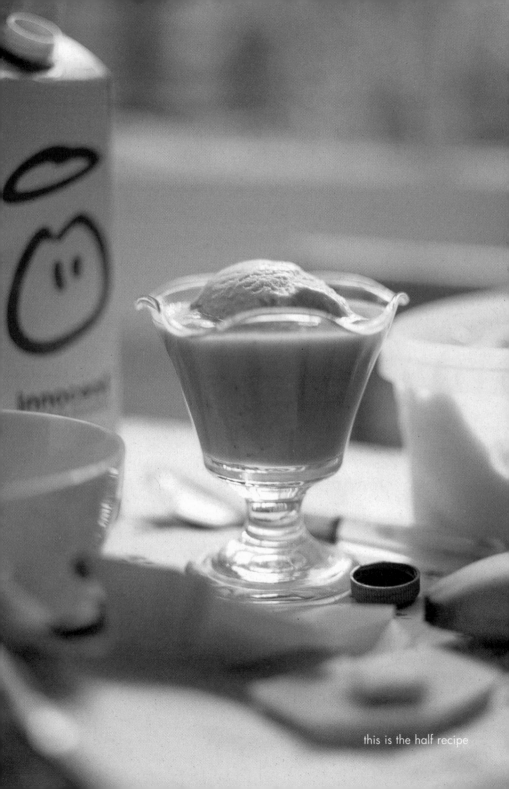

this is the half recipe

smoothie float

We have to admit that even by our standards this is a pretty lazy one to make. But you cannot deny the sheer pulling power that a bit of ice cream adds to a smoothie.

what you need
1 innocent smoothie
1 scoop of vanilla ice cream

what to do
Um, pour the smoothie into a big glass. Pop a scoop of ice cream on top. That's kind of it. 1 serving.

This works really well with our strawberries and bananas recipe.

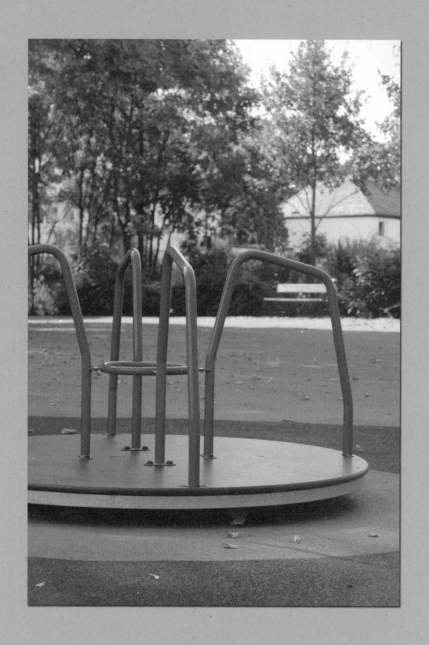

Small Wonders

**Pulling wheelies. Picking scabs.
Eating half a worm and saving the rest for later.**

These are some of the things that kids enjoy slightly
more than being told to eat fruit and veg. But there are
some mildly cunning ways to get them to eat some good
stuff. Here is a small collection of such tips:

1 It is the oldest trick – older even than the choo-choo train
method – but drawing a funny face on a plate works.
Rock solid, every time. Carrots make good noses, peas
can be arranged into mouths and here are two little
potatoes to see with.

2 Jelly and trifle are still unbeatable for pudding.
Make them even better by sneaking in some fruit
before they've set. Mango jelly is a particular favourite.

3 You wield a mighty power – the power of the lunchbox. So
please don't put rubbish into it. Dried fruit is better than a
Penguin in so many ways.

4 Set a good example. If you're turning your nose up at fruit
and veg, how are they ever going to learn? Be a brave soldier
and lead by example. And save your secret chocolate stash
until after they've gone to bed.

5 Make ice lollies from fresh fruit juice, or make some
juicy ice cubes to pop into their drinks.

6 Homemade pizzas can be topped with healthy
fresh stuff – get some pineapple on there pronto.

If you can make fruit and veg part of their everyday
life, then you've done your job. Good habits start
young. And a nutritionally balanced kid is a happy kid.

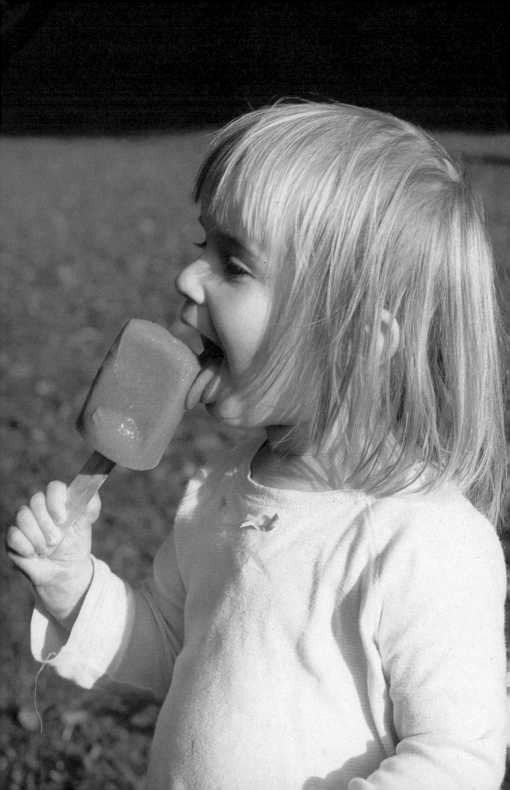

smoothie ice lollies

Another surefire way to cheat some fruit into those young people who live in your house – ice lollies.

what you need
innocent smoothies
Ice lolly moulds

what to do
Pour any innocent smoothie into ice lolly moulds and pop them into the freezer for 24 hours until frozen solid. Or freeze them using ice cube trays. Add smoothie ice cubes to brighten up boring drinks. You can get about 6 lollies from 1 smoothie.

Ice lollies were invented by the ancient Greeks, who used to suck on a Calippo whilst pondering complex philosophical questions.

lemon curd and fromage frais

We have Eleanor's mum to thank for this recipe. She made the lemon curd and came up with the idea. So we've printed the handwritten recipe she sent us on the page opposite. Thanks, Mum.

what you need
2 large apples
1 tablespoon of lemon curd
4 tablespoons of fromage frais
½ a lemon

what to do
Cut the apples into wedges, put them through the juicer and pour into the blender. Add the lemon curd, fromage frais and the zest of quarter of a lemon to the blender. Pulse twice. Don't overblend as the drink loses its body. Sprinkle some fresh lemon zest over the drink to serve. 1 greedy serving.

Useful

LEMON CURD

2 oz butter
4 oz caster sugar
1 whole egg
2 egg yolks
Finely grated rind &
juice of large organic
lemon.

Melt butter, sugar, rind
& juice in a basin in
a pan of simmering water.
Whip egg & yolks together
& strain into lemon
mixture.
Heat gently, whisking
every few
minutes until
thick (15-20 mins)
Cool & put into
jam jars.
KEEP REFRIGERATED!

what shall I drink?

The best recipe for...

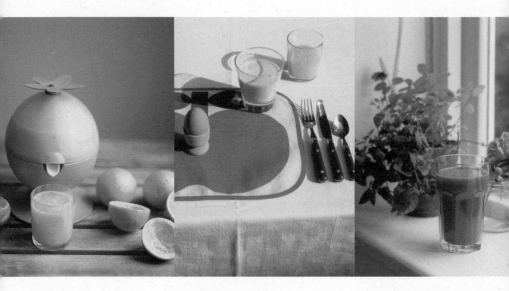

Waking you up
Orange, mango and lime 113

A liquid breakfast
Bananas, oats and medjool dates 70

Falling in love
Raspberry and roses 139

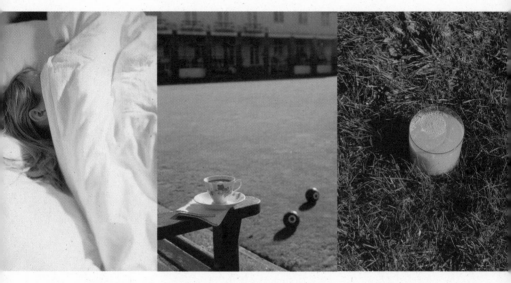

The morning after
Pomegranate and
blueberry 62

Something for your Granny
Apple, blackcurrant and
elderflower 117

Healthy glowing skin
Carrot, apple and
ginger 97

The best recipe for...

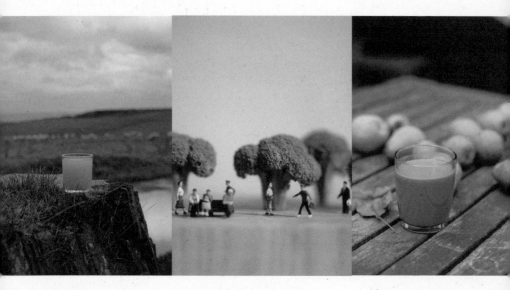

Keeping you awake at your desk on Wednesday afternoon
The Cardigan Bay Kickstart 122

Lovely pregnant ladies
Broccoli, pear and kiwi 98

Calming you down a bit
Blackberry and lavender 68

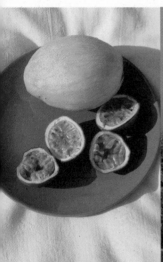 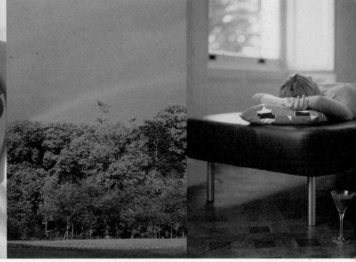

Making your hair grow
Mango and passion
fruit 28

Getting things moving
Prune and nutmeg 87

Bedtime
Dark chocolate and
cherry 145

things that are on our mind

There are quite a few issues in the world of fruit and veg that are on our mind. So we thought we'd take this chance to air them. Just think of us as that boring person having a good old drone in the snug at the Dog and Trumpet.

organic food

The organic issue occupies plenty of column inches. And rightly so – it's important for us to know the facts about the food that we eat and how it is grown or reared. But there's a bigger problem – people don't eat enough healthy stuff. We live in a nation that is only just facing up to a massive problem in the shape of obesity and heart disease. And we simply don't eat enough fruit and veg, organic or not.

So we're glad that organic food exists. It provides choice. It provides a lot of people with more of an impetus to get this healthy stuff inside them. And it's apparent that certain groups of society, such as pregnant women and the parents of young children, see the organic option as a good one.

But our main message is and always will be 'eat more fruit and veg'. Eat more natural stuff. Cram it into your diet in any way you can see fit. If the concept of eating organically makes it more likely that you'll get your five a day, that's magic. But never allow an absence of organic produce to stop you from eating fruit and veg. And please remember that eating organic doughnuts and drinking organic gin doesn't make you healthier.

food miles and local sourcing

We have more choice than ever. We can buy fruit and veg from all over the world whenever we like. But this stuff has to be transported somehow. And it's that element that has many people up in arms. According to Sustain, 'for every calorie of carrot flown in from South Africa, we use 66 calories of fuel. The huge fuel use in the food system means more carbon dioxide emissions,

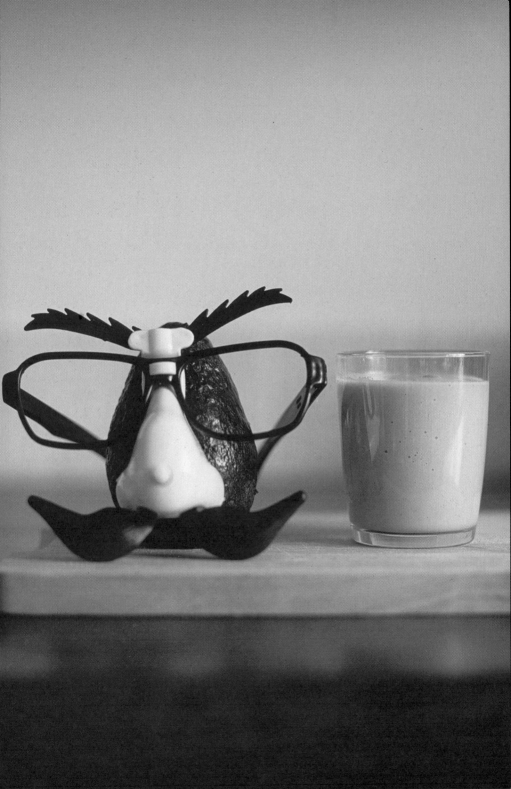

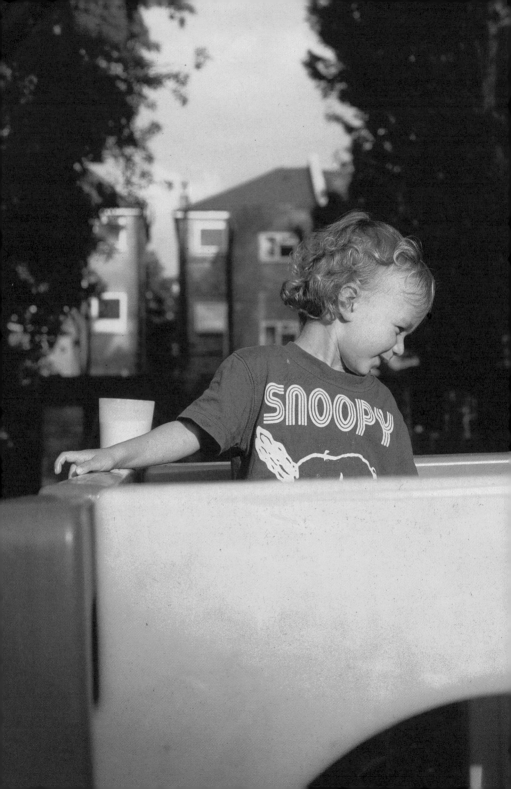

which means climate change and more damage to food supplies as well as other major health and social problems.'*

It follows that as more people become aware of this issue, the more our thoughts should turn towards sourcing locally. And it also follows that air-freight is the main culprit in this area, burning up tonnes of aviation fuel when there are more efficient ways of transporting produce.

So we have made the decision never to air-freight any of our ingredients in order to make our drinks. This can be tough, especially when we want to get the best-tasting fruit in the world, but it can be done.

And you can help too. Try to buy ingredients that are in season and check the label for the country of origin. The closer to home, the less damage you're doing. As for the holy grail, just call the local council, get yourself an allotment and grow your own. Then you'll get to fruit and veg heaven.

permed vs straight

Tough one. We like perms and we think it's about time for a perm renaissance, or 'permaissance'. But straight looks good too. It's a big decision – it's got to be your call.

*Sustain: The alliance for better food and farming – a registered charity advocating food and agriculture policies and practices that enhance the health and welfare of people and animals. http://www.sustainweb.org/about_backinfo.asp

shopping for juice – a buyer's guide

If we all had pocket-blenders, we could make our own smoothies whenever we were out and about. Unfortunately, nobody has yet made the perfect pocket-blender, and besides, they'd be quite dangerous if you were fishing around for your keys. So lots of us choose to buy ready-made smoothies and juices, which is brilliant, as long as you buy the right ones.

Here's a guide to all of the different terminology you'll encounter when buying ready-made stuff. Remember, always check the label, and always study the ingredients panel very carefully, as that's where companies are obliged by law to tell the truth.

concentrates

Concentrated juice is a juice that has been boiled, then evaporated in a vacuum and finally homogenised, resulting in a thick tar. This is then frozen, shipped to countries where it is defrosted, reconstituted with tap water and has 'add backs' added (to enhance flavour and aroma). The concentration process dramatically affects the nutritional value and the taste of the juice. We never ever use concentrates.

freshly squeezed

Fresh is best. The term 'freshly squeezed' means that the juice comes from fruit that has been brought to the UK in its natural state i.e. inside its own peel. The fruit is then squeezed locally and put into a bottle. Fresh juice has the best nutritional profile. All of our smoothies contain fresh juice.

not from concentrate (NFC)

This juice isn't freshly squeezed, but isn't a concentrate. Typically, an NFC juice is made by freezing fresh juice, shipping it and defrosting it at the other end. Lots better than a concentrate.

pasteurisation

There are two types of pasteurisation: gentle and UHT.

Gentle or flash pasteurisation is the process used on fresh milk, and for some juices. The liquid is heated for a very short period of time (3 or 4 seconds) to a moderate temperature, which doesn't affect the taste or nutritional value of the juice. All it does is knock out the bugs that make juice go 'off', and it's also an important health safeguard. In the 1990s an outbreak of e-coli in the USA was traced to a smoothie company that didn't pasteurise its juices, leading to the death of one person. In the USA, if you don't pasteurise your juice, you are obliged to place a health warning on your label.

UHT (ultra heat treatment) pasteurisation is the process that produces long-life milk. It's used to remove anything that could cause the product to go off, meaning that the carton or bottle can sit on the (unrefrigerated) shelf for months. As you might imagine, these drinks aren't very nutritious, having been subjected to extreme temperatures for a long period of time. We say avoid.

pure/100% fruit

There is nothing in this product apart from juice. However, the drink may not be fresh, it could be NFC or it could contain concentrates. Check the ingredients panel thoroughly to find out.

smoothie

A proper smoothie is a blend of whole crushed fruit and freshly squeezed juices. It should not contain any added sugar or water and should most importantly be made with fresh rather than concentrated juices. Naturally, it should also be free of any weird additives, and will always be thicker and more pulpy than a normal fruit juice.

thickie

A blend of probiotic yoghurt, fruit, honey and spices. We made this name up in 1999 and are still waiting for it to catch on.

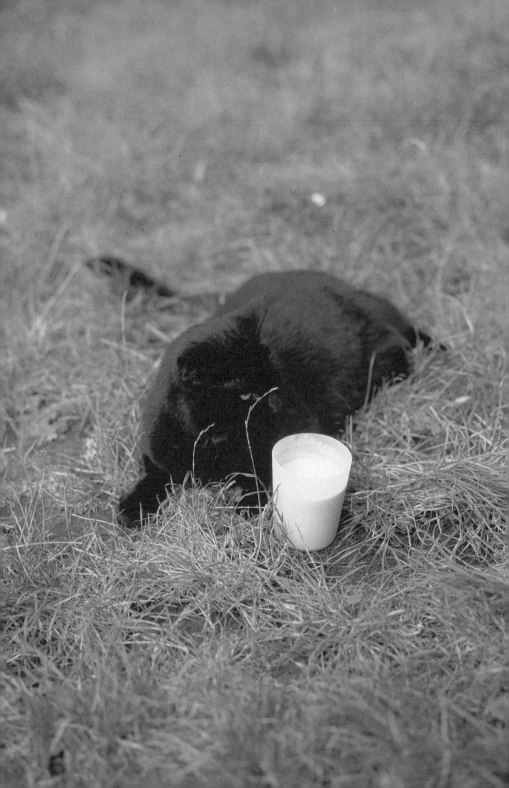

thanks

thanks for the recipes

Wow. We wrote another book. And the recipes are our best yet. So the biggest thanks are reserved for our innocent recipe inventors – Lucy E, Lucy T, Nikki, Amy, Eleanor and Sarah.

And then there are our guest recipe inventors – Scania and David at howies, Micah at Green & Black's, Allegra at Leon, Lizzie at Baby Organix and Jamie Oliver. Thanks for taking the time to think up nice drinks.

We can't forget all of the innocent drinkers who sent in recipes for us to choose from. Sorry we couldn't fit you all in. We chose our favourite five: Jo and Andrew, Debbie, Guni, Natasha and Paul. Hats off to you all.

And thanks to Karen for testing all of the recipes and for getting up early to find the best fruit at the market.

thanks for the design and photos

Joby made the book look hot and showed us his grid. Ed and Kat crafted beautiful interruptions (the bits that aren't recipes) along with Joby. Rachel and Julian took our mess and made everything look slick.

And Clare took some magnificent photos. They're beautiful.

Our models included our friends Hannah, Sara, Oscar, Sarah, Tessa, Stella and Elvis the cat.

Other thanks go to Daphne at Greenpeace for the picture, our mystery man at NASA, Clare and David for housing us when we went to Wales, Stacy (aged 11) for her trampoline picture and the Shrimp for keeping an eye on things.

thanks for the guidance

Louise, Julian and especially Silvia, without whom there wouldn't be a book.

thank you

The biggest 'thanks' goes to everyone who buys our drinks. We wouldn't be here without you. If you want to stay in touch, join the family at www.innocentdrinks.co.uk/family

And if you fancy working here, try www.innocentdrinks.co.uk/jobs

index